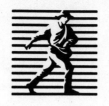

THE DIET-TYPE WEIGHT-LOSS PROGRAM

Ronald L. Hoffman, M.D.

Simon and Schuster

New York   London   Toronto   Sydney   Tokyo

Published by Simon and Schuster
A Division of Simon & Schuster Inc.
Simon & Schuster Building
Rockefeller Center
1230 Avenue of the Americas
New York, NY 10020

SIMON AND SCHUSTER and colophon are registered trademarks of
Simon & Schuster Inc.

Designed by Beth Tondreau Design / Carol Barr
Manufactured in the United States of America

10 9 8 7 6 5 4 3 2 1

Library of Congress Cataloging-in-Publication Data

Hoffman, Ronald L.
   The diet-type weight-loss program / Ronald L. Hoffman.
   p.   cm.
   Includes index.
   1. Reducing diets. I. Title.
RM222.2.H576   1988
613.2′5—dc19   88-6684
                                                                   CIP

ISBN 0-671-64642-7

ACKNOWLEDGMENTS

My special gratitude to Denise Fortino for her invaluable help with this book; to Craig Hollander, whose culinary expertise is reflected in the recipes; and to Heidi Meyer-Bothling for her able technical assistance. Thanks as well to the staff of the Whole Life Medical Center, a living laboratory for the principles in these pages. And finally, loving acknowledgment to my wife, Helen, whose support and encouragement were indispensable.

CONTENTS

I

WHAT'S YOUR DIET TYPE?

1

SETTING THE STAGE

Yes, You Have a Diet Type

Imagine this: A man and a woman, unknown to one another, visit the same doctor on the same day, each complaining of a chronic headache. In both cases, the physician takes a careful medical history and checks his patient's heart rate, blood pressure and other vital signs for clues. While their outward symptoms are almost identical—a pounding sensation near the temples and sides of the head—very little else about them is. For example, the man, a portly retired salesman in his sixties, drinks heavily and leads a sedentary life; the woman, a professional dancer in her twenties, is petite, wiry, athletic and always under pressure to perform. The disorders that run in their families are very different, as are the results of their most recent physical examinations. It is no wonder, then, that the advice and prescriptions they receive turn out to be markedly different, too.

If "doctor's orders" can vary widely from person to person, even for those with the very same complaints, why shouldn't a "prescription" for dieting? When it comes to weight loss, people are definitely *not* alike. They differ in the rate at which they gain and lose pounds, as well as in where they accumulate them, when, and the reasons they become and stay overweight. Even more important, they have distinct eating habits, preferences, life-styles, medical histories and attitudes toward food that will determine the kind of diet that suits them best. *No single eating plan or set of strategies can serve everyone's needs.*

Some diets, however wholesome or effective, make impractical demands on a person's daily routine, culinary tastes or beliefs, or are ill-matched to certain behavior. For example, if you tend to binge or nibble throughout the day, you may feel restricted by a three-meals-a-day-only format. You may be a heavy eater, accustomed to large quantities of food, or reluctant to give up meat; salads, sprouts and tofu just won't do it for you. If you work long hours or travel and entertain clients a lot, you may be unwilling or unable to shop for certain foods or prepare them a special way. Back home, you prefer to have a quick take-out meal or to heat up some frozen entree since you are so pressed for time. Your friend may have had success with a given regimen, but when you try it you can't even budge the scale. Or you lose just as much weight as he or she did, but you feel terribly hungry or fatigued as a result.

About two months before she came to see me, one of my patients had started enthusiastically on a famous, best-selling diet. To her delight, she had begun losing weight fairly steadily, just as the program promised, but soon after, she noticed a feeling she had never experienced before: morning sluggishness and lethargy, even occasional nausea. "I'd always been an early riser, bright-eyed and wide awake by seven, but suddenly I didn't seem to have any energy at all —at least until mid-afternoon," Andrea recalled.

The diet she was on permitted only fruit until noon, then later added proteins and carbohydrates, separately. When I tested Andrea, she turned out to be extremely intolerant of sugar: In response to a specially supervised "stimulus" meal of mostly fruit, her blood glucose level rose sharply, then dropped way down. And that is exactly what happened when she was on the fruit (sugar) portion of her diet—she felt completely wiped out in a matter of minutes. "Some of my friends *swear* by this diet," she said, "and I lost weight with it, too. But unlike them, I feel tired all the time. That's why I've come looking for another answer."

Too many diets, especially those that don't fit the dieter, deliver only short-term results, and, what's more, the search for slimness can become progressively self-defeating. Take the case of Suzanne, the thirty-eight-year old admitted "diet pro" who for the past twenty years had been losing weight "successfully" on almost every popular plan imaginable. Trouble was, she invariably gained those pounds back (an all too common phenomenon!). When she came to me, she had gotten stuck at the 185-to-190-pound mark and was finding it increasingly hard to slim down yet again. "Put me on a diet and I'll follow it to the letter," she observed. "But once the two or three weeks are up, or I see a food that's not on the 'permitted' list, I start to *panic*. Without the structure of a disciplined menu, I feel lost, out of control. How do I keep going? How can I trust myself once a diet is finished?"

To skip ahead a few steps, Suzanne is now a gorgeous, healthy 132 pounds and has stayed that way for several years —an excellent sign. (It's fair to describe a diet as successful only if a person stays within 10 percent of his or her new weight after five years or more.) For now, I will say only that we got her to look at food in an entirely new way—as part of an ongoing life-style rather than a restricted two-or-three-week diet with a clear-cut beginning, middle and end.

But the story does not finish here. While Suzanne apparently thrived on her mostly complex-carbohydrate meals, Mark, a corporate executive whom I initially treated in exactly the same way, did not. His body did not respond well to too many whole grains or starchy vegetables. They caused him to gain rather than lose weight, because he is what I call "carbohydrate sensitive." He also found it too time-consuming to shop for and prepare some of the suggested menus. Mark obviously required—and received—a very different approach from Suzanne's—and that is the whole point: One person's ideal diet can be another person's disaster.

Because it limits the amount of food you eat by regulating portions or banning certain items, almost *any* diet, no matter how awful or admirable, will do the trick—for a while. But if it is not compatible with your personal habits and hang-ups, your life-style and body chemistry, and if it fails to reinforce healthful patterns of eating and relating to food, it will not keep its promise. No matter that your friend or sister or coworker may have had great results on one or another program. If you have not, it is because of important differences between you and them, and not a deficiency of luck or discipline. In short, you have not failed, but rather *your diet has failed you.* Remember, the story of weight loss contains no complicated plot twists or major mysteries. With a way of eating and living that truly fits your personal profile, you can lose body fat, keep it off and stay healthy for a lifetime.

To find a diet you can live with, you must first evaluate your needs and goals and discover where you belong in the diet scheme. Through the carefully designed multipart self-test in Chapter 3, composed of a series of questions similar to the ones I use in my daily practice, you will be able to identify your diet history, peeves and preferences, daily routines, personality traits, attitudes, medical conditions and other variables and ultimately match yourself up with the diet most compatible for you.

Some portions of the self-appraisal test will serve an important psychological function by encouraging you to think about yourself. For example, you might become aware, perhaps for the very first time, of such basics as how much or how often you eat, the habits or moods that accompany these occasions and the easily overlooked ways in which you may keep sabotaging your efforts. You might also discover that you have some strictly physical or inherited disadvantages that have made it a bit harder for you to stay slim (see Chapter 2). Whatever the case, once you learn why weight loss has been a challenge for you in the past, you can redirect your energies for better results.

The rewards of changing your relationship to food may reach far beyond appearances. If you are between twenty and thirty and are even moderately overweight (about 10 or 20 percent above the ideal weight for your height and build), you are at higher risk for heart disease in later years and have a shorter-than-average life expectancy. If you are under forty-five, you are also a more likely candidate for high blood pressure, diabetes and elevated blood cholesterol, along with gallstones, respiratory disorders and degenerative changes in the joints, particularly the knees and hips. (Apparently, weight gained in early adulthood is associated with greater health risks than that acquired later in life.)

Overweight women have a greater chance of developing malignant tumors of the ovaries and uterine lining and, after menopause, of the breasts. Obese men have a higher incidence of certain cancers, including those of the colon, rectum and prostate.

While no one can guarantee that dieting away a given quantity of fat will add a specific number of years to your life, losing even small amounts of weight can directly lower cholesterol and blood pressure and regulate diabetes.

But even if you are not overweight, you can court all these ills and more if you eat unwisely. Leanness itself is no guarantee of superior health if your food calories are from the wrong sources. Fortunately, more of us are getting the message: We want to eat sensibly, not only to look good and to lose 10 or 20 pounds, but also to feel better, live longer, have more vigor and energy. Growing numbers of us are exercising regularly and reducing our intake of meats while increasing our consumption of whole grains, fresh vegetables and fruits. We are more aware that eating for slimness and high nutrition are inseparable, and that both must be lifetime propositions. For this reason, *The Diet-Type Weight-Loss Program* is intended not just for dieters, but also for the countless people of normal weight who are seeking a prescription for lasting health.

THE FIVE DIET TYPES

To use a simple analogy, just as everyone has a blood type and a skin type, so he or she also has a diet type. Based on years of research and clinical experience with over 100 patients a week, I have found that each of us is best served by any one of five basic diet categories, which I have labeled as follows: 1. The High-Fiber/Super Grain Diet; 2. The Modified Protein-Plus Diet; 3. The No-More-Allergies Diet; 4. The Natural Raw Foods Diet and 5. The Bored of Health Diet.

Each of these approaches, adopted for life, can be highly beneficial for certain people, depending on their physical and emotional makeup, and each has its own set of advantages and drawbacks. My purpose is to reinforce the positive features of all five Diet Types so that no matter what your ideal choice, you can be assured of excellent results for both your appearance and your health.

When I first started treating the overweight, I thought that one kind of diet could work for everyone and that people just had to be properly educated and converted to this one true way of eating. But my medical experience has taught me that, for any number of reasons, not everyone thrives on one such regimen, and it is necessary to offer people variations on this basic theme—wholesome, well-conceived alternatives that better serve the body's or the psyche's needs.

The only way to step off the diet treadmill and rescue yourself from a less-than-perfect state of health is to know what weight-loss alternatives are possible, how they work and what *you* respond to best. Each of the five basic Diet Types emphasizes particular categories of foods and is designed for certain needs and life-styles. In addition, a number of guidelines and strategies, essential to the success of any diet, are aimed at altering your eating behavior. These points, which cover getting started, progressing past a "plateau" and maintaining hard-won results, are featured in Chapter 9 and are relevant to all the Diet Types. They will help ensure a good behavioral match between you and whatever Diet Type you ultimately choose.

Below are brief capsule descriptions of the five basic Diet Types and their special features:

DIET TYPE 1: The High-Fiber/Super Grain Diet

You can actually eat more and weigh less on this diet —no strict portion control is required! Plentiful in complex carbohydrates—whole grains, cereals, pasta, potatoes, legumes, fresh vegetables and fruits—low in fat and featuring far more protein from plant than animal sources, this way of eating has a marvelous track record for safe, steady weight loss as well as protection from heart disease, cancer, diabetes and other serious conditions. Along with all the other Diet Types, it will be described in much greater detail in Part II.

DIET TYPE 2: The Modified Protein-Plus Diet

This diet is designed for those who wish to take advantage of an effective weight-loss plan that features their favorite protein foods and healthful, lower-fat alternatives. It is well suited to restaurant eating and traditional gourmet recipes, and may be helpful for certain medical conditions. It may also benefit those who crave carbohydrates and wind up bingeing on them at every opportunity. By downplaying some carbohydrates, the Modified Protein Plan can help you avoid the foods that tempt you to overeat.

DIET TYPE 3: The No-More-Allergies Diet

Some people do not digest certain carbohydrates well and may react with gassiness and bloating, or even outright allergic symptoms, particularly to wheat or milk products. For them, Diet Type 3 may be the answer. It is aimed at those who either crave or respond unfavorably to certain foods and whose chronic symptoms may result from diagnosed or suspected allergies. By "rotating" troublesome items—carefully timing when they are eaten—it helps break the food sensitivities and dependencies that lead to unwanted weight gain in some people. Even if you are in a strictly psychological rut, this plan can show you how to add greater variety and flexibility to your meals.

DIET TYPE 4: *The Natural Raw Foods Diet*

This eating plan emphasizes carbohydrates in the form of leafy greens (raw or lightly cooked) and fresh fruits instead of whole grains and starchy vegetables. It is a predominantly vegetarian diet, high in water content, vitamins, minerals, enzymes and fiber. Light, refreshing and easy to prepare, the menus are a natural for spring and summer or warm climates all year round. Some versions of this diet have stressed "food combining," a now discredited principle regulating the order and combinations in which foods may be eaten. Following a certain sequence is *not* necessary for this diet to work, with very few exceptions, which I will explain in detail in Chapter 7. Since it is so low in sodium and fat and high in potassium, the Raw Foods Diet is excellent for those with hypertension, high blood cholesterol or a family history of heart disease; people with arthritis and psoriasis have responded quite well to it, too.

DIET TYPE 5: *The Bored of Health Diet*

This program aims to build on the best in the American diet and tends more to the mainstream than the exotic. For those short on time or patience (or both), the plan serves up supermarket food, often of the ready-made variety, and is also easy to follow on the road, where standard restaurant/hotel fare is common. The challenge for me as a physician was to design a series of all-American meals that were nutritionally high-powered yet also responsibly low in sodium, fat and cholesterol, the traditional "terrible trio" of our country's cuisine. The growing number of innovative "lite" food products and the increasing emphasis on more wholesome ingredients—even take-out delis and fast-food outlets feature such items now—made my task easier.

Selecting from a variety of Diet Types that reflect a wide range of tastes and approaches is a timely concept, since choice has become the rule among health-minded eaters. Today's style of dieting is far more flexible than fanatic, with purists and pleasure-seekers alike aiming toward a middle ground. Strict health-food types show signs of becoming more relaxed, too. *The New York Times* recently reported that some otherwise conscientious folks have been allowing themselves more meat, ice cream, pizza and candy in recent years. They have also been buying more walking than running shoes, and switching to the softer, low-impact kind of aerobics. In short, they have been easing up on the absolutist, obsessive approach to nutrition and fitness.

At the same time, Americans are showing greater interest in vegetarian-based cuisines without necessarily becoming full-fledged converts. The consumption of fresh vegetables is up 12 percent since 1980. Middle Eastern, Indian and Mexican restaurants, which feature grains and beans, have become more popular. Those with newfound reverence for vegetables who still pile their plates with chicken and fish are proudly describing themselves as "polyvegetarians." Even the most casual eaters and diehard red-meat fans are demanding and buying more "lite" alternatives—lower in fat, salt, sugar, cholesterol and other undesirables. It is becoming trendy to eat healthy, to have more vegetables and grains, to indulge in smaller portions of familiar fatty favorites. The ultra-lean 3-ounce steak is fast replacing the well-marbled 16-ounce variety. It is also easier to find nonmeat meals at elegant restaurants.

What can we make of all this? People on all sides of the diet spectrum are experimenting with alternative ways of eating, showing more flexibility and allowing for greater variety in their own meals. They are interested in eating for pleasure as well as protection from serious disease, including obesity. Most important, they are trying to find their own place in the diet scheme and are confirming the need for individual choices instead of following one diet "ideology" designed for all.

DESPERATE MEASURES

While more people are eating better, we still have a long way to go. According to a recent government survey, nearly 34 million adult Americans—or 26 percent of adults between twenty and seventy-five—are overweight, and more than 12 million of them are substantially so. Too many are *diet desperate,* searching for the ultimate one-step breakthrough, and the weight-loss business flourishes as never before. Last year, Americans spent some $200 million on over-the-counter diet drugs and amphetamine-related compounds, and millions more for special powder and liquid formulas and nonsensical natural remedies like kelp and grapefruit extract. There was, in addition, the usual avalanche of popular, promise-all diet plans. The lure of such approaches is that of the proverbial easy way out, the classic quick fix—and what dieter can resist the temptation? It is no secret that medical doctors and other professionals have traditionally failed to provide their patients with effective nutrition/weight-loss counseling. Since they have not adequately addressed this need, they must share at least some of the blame for those who do so irresponsibly. Without proper guidance, dieters cannot evaluate the many claims put before them. More unscientific, unhealthy and even dangerous solutions to obesity are touted than to any other medical problem.

Unfortunately, being seduced by artful promises can become a lifetime habit. Suzanne, the self-described "diet pro," is an all too common case, graduating from one shortsighted diet to another in an increasingly futile search for slimness. When you diet the wrong way, persistence does *not* pay off: The more often you try to lose weight, the harder it becomes to do it. The reason, in brief, is that when you sharply cut back its food supply, the body responds defensively, as if it were gearing up for starvation or a serious energy deficit. To protect itself, it starts using up its energy more slowly— which means that it does not burn off calories as readily to carry on its normal functions (see Chapter 2). Thus, with each successive diet, it becomes more difficult to lose pounds on the same amount of food. You have to "starve" your body further to see results—and it will defend itself more vigorously every time (the classic vicious circle!). Years of repeated, rapid dieting take their toll not only on your health but also on your capacity for effective weight loss. This ironic condition has been called "diet-induced obesity." No wonder many doctors have said it is better not to lose weight at all than to make a habit of it.

RELAX!

I have often found that those who are most preoccupied with dieting have the greatest difficulty reaching their goals and are the most frequent victims of "diet-induced obesity." I advise them to focus on *health* as their primary concern, which eliminates the pressure of having to lose a certain number of pounds in a given period of time. Think of the insomniac who gets better results by relaxing with a glass of warm milk instead of willing himself to sleep. Become obsessed with staying fit, energetic and immune to disease, rather than with the scale—and weight loss will naturally follow!

The presence of so many Suzannes is evidence enough that huge numbers of people have been subsisting on a steady diet of misinformation. Indeed, with all the diet data currently in the air, many of us are simply confused, unable to synthesize the wealth of news and advice, to separate fact from myth and apply it to our own lives. Even the best-informed may be armed largely with half-truths and partial know-how, vague ideas and educated guesses when it comes to dieting and nutrition. Those of us who *are* well versed and are already following a reasonable diet may wish to refine or modify the program, or find out whether it is the ideal choice.

Presenting the state-of-the-art essentials, the next chapter will help you understand why you are overweight and show you the very best ways of confronting it. It will give you the information you need to evaluate the weight-loss alternatives available to you and where you belong among them. And it will make you a more sophisticated, harder-to-fool consumer who can better distinguish bogus claims from bona fide information.

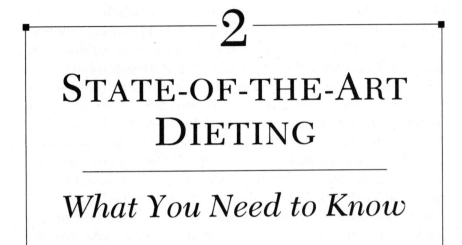

STATE-OF-THE-ART DIETING

What You Need to Know

Forget much of what you have learned up to now about the rules of dieting—conventional weight-loss wisdom has been radically revised. To begin with, the fine art of counting calories turns out to be mostly a waste of time. Dieters and nutritionists alike once believed that losing weight was simply a matter of staying off balance for a while, expending more calories than you took in through food. As long as you stayed within a certain calorie limit or burned up sufficient energy, you'd be assured of a slimmer body. But as most of us discovered on our own, the arithmetic never held up well in practice. We may have written off our diet failures as proof of a character flaw or a lapse in discipline, but scientists today know better.

If you eat a 500 calorie meal, for example, it matters very much where those calories are coming from—fats, proteins or carbohydrates—because the body handles each of them quite differently. Just tallying up the numbers is not enough.

While overindulging in *any* kind of food can lead to weight gain, the surplus fat in our diets is a more likely source of trouble than an abundance of either complex carbohydrates or lean proteins. It's when refined, sugary carbohydrates are linked with fats, as in ice cream, cakes and pastries, or when proteins are liberally accompanied by fats, as in hamburgers, bacon, sausage and cheese, that they may threaten both your weight and health. Still designed for prehistoric times, when famine was a common threat, the human body is programmed to *store* fat—its emergency backup fuel—and to *burn* carbohydrates for immediate energy. (It uses up protein primarily to repair and maintain its tissues.) What's more, our fat-storing capacity is virtually unlimited. Regardless of how many fat cells we have (see below), they seem capable of accommodating an endless supply of fat. By contrast, we can pack away only a limited amount of reserve carbohydrate energy, known as glycogen, in our muscles, and only a small percentage of it can be *readily* turned into fat. Unlike most carbohydrates in their natural state, fat is also easy to overeat, because it does not contain stomach-filling bulk.

The moral for dieters: don't focus on calories; it's their quality, not quantity, that counts above all. Do cut back on fats. And bear in mind that it's hard to gain weight on unrefined, complex carbohydrates—whole grains, legumes, fresh vegetables and fruits—so you should definitely be paying more attention to these foods, no matter what your chosen diet. They will stick to your ribs, but not to your body!

Another practice being questioned by today's dieting know-how is that of weighing in on the bathroom scale. Here, too, the numbers alone tell a very sketchy story. Just as with calories, all pounds—and all fat cells—are not alike. It's the kind, size and quantity of fat cells and the way they're distributed throughout the body that are crucial. Most overweight people don't have *more* fat cells than everyone else, but larger ones that expand more easily. (Only people who are 60 percent or more above their normal weight are believed to be burdened with a greater-than-average number of fat cells.)

More important, fat cells *behave* differently depending on their makeup. All 40-odd billion of them contain both alpha- and beta-receptors, which act to synthesize and break down

ALL CALORIES ARE NOT ALIKE

Beware: Fat is the most *concentrated* food you can eat. Just one gram of it supplies 9 calories, compared to 4 for the same amount of carbohydrate or protein. In fact, a recent study by Mark Hegsted, a noted professor of nutrition at the Harvard School of Public Health, found that fat may be "worth" as much as 11 calories per gram, or almost three times as much as protein or carbohydrate! He and other researchers have concluded that the fat in our diets is more easily converted into body fat than is any other kind of food.

What's more, a Swiss study found that when we eat fat, the body burns only 3 percent of its calories to store it. But packing away the same amount of carbohydrate uses up 23 percent of the calories from a meal. Since it doesn't come naturally, storing carbohydrate takes more of a toll. Of course, the body prefers the much easier job of retaining fat—which is why you'll gain more weight from a high-fat meal than a low-fat one, even if they add up to the same number of calories.

fats, respectively. Thus, the alpha areas of the cell are designed to take in fatty acids and promote weight gain, while the beta regions more easily burn stored fat when the body requires energy. These two functions take place simultaneously. However, the cells that are alpha-dominant further the buildup and storage of fat, while the beta-dominant cells encourage its release. Generally, men tend to have more of their fat-retaining cells in the abdomen and stomach, while women are more apt to have them in their hips, thighs and buttocks. This explains why men are often prone to accumulate fat around the middle, giving them a potbellied, or "apple," shape, and why many women are troubled by a bottom-heavy, or "pear-shaped," look. The female hormones estrogen and progesterone appear to dictate this pattern of fat distribution, particularly during a woman's childbearing years, to provide potential support and "cushioning" for a developing fetus.

Thus, each sex has its vulnerable zone where excess weight is most visible and resistant to the effects of dieting. On the one hand, apples may be somewhat luckier, since the abdomen and stomach are believed to be armed with more beta-receptors than are the tissues below the waist, allowing for easier weight loss. However, round-the-middle fat, even in an otherwise slim individual, is also associated with an alarmingly higher risk of heart disease, atherosclerosis, hypertension, diabetes, ovarian cancer and early death. While extra padding on hips, thighs and rear may not match the Hollywood ideal, it's a lot safer to carry around.

Another type of adipose tissue, called "brown fat," which makes up about 1 percent of your body weight, is capable of burning large amounts of energy. These specialized fat cells apparently thrive on vigorous exercise. Along with a diet rich in carbohydrates, physical activity stimulates them to produce great quantities of heat, which accelerates weight loss. In yet another nod to biochemistry, some scientists believe that a number of overweight people may have sluggish or nonfunctioning brown fat cells.

Obviously, the shape of your body and the type and arrangement of your fat cells will help determine how fast you lose weight (as well as how prone you are to certain diseases.) That's why two people who weigh exactly the same amount at the start of a diet can end up with very different results even if they have identical eating and exercise habits.

Understanding fat-cell behavior helps make it clear why repeated dieting can make you fat. The following may have happened to you: After trying several diets, each time losing several pounds and then gaining them back, you notice that with each new effort it takes you longer to lose and a lot less

FAT CELLS AT A GLANCE

	Alpha	*Beta*
EXERCISE (AEROBIC)		triggers their release
BINGEING/LARGE MEALS	stimulates their enlargement	
DISTRIBUTION IN WOMEN	hips, thighs, buttocks	stomach, upper body
DISTRIBUTION IN MEN	stomach, upper body	hips, thighs, buttocks
FUNCTION	cushioning, fat depots	source of ready energy
HEALTH RISKS	serious when predominant in stomach, upper body	none
EASE OF WEIGHT LOSS	difficult	easy

time to revert to your former weight. Curbing your food intake on each occasion awakens your body's ancient "famine control" center. The fat cells, perceiving the shortage of food as a threat, start taking steps to ensure their survival. For example, the once-generous beta cells begin withholding their stores of fat and the brain receives signals to slow down the body's metabolism (the rate at which it burns calories and eliminates excess weight).

The level of weight below which your body refuses to budge is known as your *setpoint*. This "bottom line" is believed to be genetically determined, although many factors can push it up or down. A fat-rich diet, pregnancy (high levels of estrogen and progesterone are friendly to alpha cells) and advancing age can raise the setpoint; consistent aerobic exercise is one effective way of lowering it (see below). Bear in mind that the setpoint doesn't discriminate. Some very thin people have reported just as much frustration trying to *gain* weight; their bodies speed up the metabolic tempo when they eat high-calorie meals, thus canceling out any surplus.

To illustrate how persistent your fat cells are: in a Rockefeller University experiment, a group of rats were fed barely enough to keep them alive. After a month, once their bodies had used up all their extra fat reserves, they started consuming their own muscle and connective tissue—but both their fat cells and brain cells still remained intact. Our persevering, well-protected fat cells are part of the survival mechanism held over from our past history, when periodic starvation was the rule. I tell my overweight patients that

START YOUNG

The earlier you manage weight, the better. Fat acquired during childhood is believed to increase the body's total number of fat cells, especially the acquisitive alpha kind. Fat gained later in life tends to settle in the abdomen and middle, where it may be easier to lose. This means that preventing childhood obesity would go a long way toward overcoming the problem once and for all.

their bodies are superbly adapted to such a crisis, and that they would surely survive a severe, long-term food shortage, whereas I probably would not! Unfortunately, in affluent, food-abundant countries like ours, what was once a sign of biological superiority and a distinct survival advantage is now simply a serious health liability.

IS THERE A FAT GENE?

Heredity can be a powerful factor in deciding our size and shape, influencing how easily we gain or lose weight. A study of 540 adults who had been adopted as children found that their weight in each case more closely resembled that of their biological rather than their adoptive parents. And scientists have already calculated that if both your parents are overweight, your chances of following suit are 80 percent, compared to a 14 percent chance of becoming overweight if you have two parents of normal weight.

However, genes do *not* determine weight the same way they do skin, hair or eye color. You may be predisposed to gain weight, but only your diet and eating behavior can make it happen. Also, keep in mind that identical twins remain close in weight until puberty, when environment becomes the more compelling factor.

SLOW DOWN—AND GET MOVING!

On a quick-weight-loss diet, which is typically very high in protein and low in carbohydrates, the body is forced to draw on its stored carbohyrates, or glycogen, for energy. This power supply, in solution with water, is found in both the muscles and liver. However, if few ready carbohydrates are available in the diet, these glycogen reserves are soon exhausted, and the body must then turn to two other sources of stored calories: fat and protein. Ironically, the burning of stored fat requires some minimal amounts of carbohydrates, to prime the metabolic pump, so to speak. Thus, carbohydrate deficit also means that fat cannot be properly utilized, which leaves the body no choice but to make fuel (glucose) out of its stored muscle and structural protein tissue by a process called "gluconeogenesis." As you diet in any "crash" or unbalanced way at the expense of carbohydrates, you rapidly run out of stored glycogen and consequently lose a lot of lean muscle tissue, along with some fat and a good deal of water.

Once you go off the quick-fix diet and begin eating normally again, chances are you'll gain back the lost pounds, and then some. Remember, your body, acting in self-defense, has already slowed down its energy-burning rate, which means it requires fewer calories to keep all systems running than it did before. Thus, "normal" eating will represent *more* than what your body needs, and can easily turn into extra weight. Worse, the pounds will return largely in the form of fat, rather than lean muscle. Since you have already lost a disproportionate amount of muscle compared to fat, this is especially bad news. With each diet "rebound," your body contours will actually change (even if your actual weight does not), making you look flabbier than before. It also takes less food energy to sustain fat than muscle, so you won't have to eat that much to stay out of shape!

Apparently, the more sedentary you are, the more lean muscle you lose. A study reported in *The American Journal of Clinical Nutrition* put eight women hospitalized for obesity on a strictly controlled, 800-calorie diet for five weeks. Five of the volunteers participated in a supervised program of daily aerobic exercise and three of them remained inactive. The total weight loss was, somewhat surprisingly, not very different between the exercising and nonexercising groups. However, significantly more of the loss came from fat and less from lean muscle mass in the women who worked out.

Exercise must be truly aerobic to have any slimming benefits, because the body's fat cells require ample oxygen to burn their stored fats. Short, intensive bursts of activity such as sprints use up carbohydrates but don't deliver enough oxygen to allow the body's fat-burning furnace to work.

Scientists have known for some time about the "afterglow" of aerobic exercise—how it helps the body release calories faster for up to several hours after an activity. In a recent study at Stanford University, the benefits of vigorous activity were convincingly reconfirmed. Volunteers who jogged twelve miles a week continued to burn calories and lose weight steadily even when they increased their food intake (by up to 400 calories a day) and kept exercising at the same level. What's more, the ratio of their HDLs, or "good" cholesterol, to their LDLs, the "bad" kind, increased substantially.

If you eat sensibly you can certainly lose weight, but if you do so without exercising aerobically, you will just as certainly have trouble keeping it off. A sustained twenty-five to forty-five minutes' worth of activity at least three or four times a week will help you achieve lasting results by preventing weight rebound. The newest research suggests that low-impact aerobics or the "effortless" kind done in water (hydroaerobics) may actually burn fat most efficiently. Though more carbohydrate calories are burned in a tough, sweaty workout, the body's fat stores are released more readily the *longer-lasting* and *less demanding* the exercise. Thus, crawl swimming, cycling and brisk walking are excellent aerobic choices, and distance running is preferable to racing if you're trying to trim away excess flab.

Whether you're sedentary or not, rapid dieting exacts a heavy toll. When weight loss exceeds just half a pound a day, the extra loss is bound to be lean body mass, not fat. You may also experience fatigue, loss of strength and endurance, changes in skin texture, hair loss and even depression.

Obviously, you don't have to overeat to put on weight—

dieting the wrong way can have the same result! In fact, studies have shown that a majority of the overweight *eat no more* than their normal-weight peers.

In cases where someone's appetite *is* out of bounds, biochemistry, once again, may supply the reason. After a meal, the body releases insulin into the bloodstream to process the glucose from foods and allow it to be utilized by the cells. The insulin then enters the spinal fluid, and when it reaches a certain level, it gains access to the brain and relays the message that you're full. In some overweight people, the insulin supply may be inadequate, or (because of "insulin resistance") it may take considerably longer for the hormone to be released and to reach the brain, so the satisfaction signal is delayed and they don't stop eating as quickly.

People who always find themselves struggling to control their food cravings may also have low levels of the brain chemical serotonin, which is associated with feelings of fullness. Others may produce higher-than-normal amounts of the enzyme LPL (lipoprotein lipase), which promotes fat storage and fat-cell expansion. Most important, repeated dieting is believed to stimulate this response.

While all this sounds fairly hopeless, behavior can outwit biology. Try to determine where you fit in the scenario so far. If you're the graduate of many short-term diets and have rebounded more than once, you'll know enough to avoid the same kind of eating plan. If you have more weight in the lower part of your body, you won't blame yourself if you don't slim down as quickly as your apple-shaped friend. You'll also be vigilant if one or both your parents is carrying extra weight.

How can you escape the diet-go-round? Begin by reducing as much of your body fat as possible—to a point you can reach with relative ease, before your body starts resisting, or leveling off. Remember, do this by curbing fat intake but not by *undereating,* which will only arouse your body's defenses. (All the Diet Types allow for moderate, not drastically restricted, amounts of food.)

Eating large amounts of food in one sitting, or bingeing, stimulates tenacious alpha fat cells to multiply—and the more you have, the harder it is to lose weight. To keep fat cells under control, have three square meals or more frequent, smaller ones throughout the day.

Using the menus on your chosen Diet Type as your guide, keep portions of meals and snacks roughly the suggested sizes until this way of eating becomes second nature to you. And read Chapter 9, which covers strategies that can reinforce the results of any diet and be implemented for a lifetime.

Along with smart eating, vigorous exercise that works the heart and lungs and the large muscle groups is the most effective way to lower your setpoint. Exercise preserves and even increases muscle tissue as it stimulates the body-trimming beta and brown fat cells. As already noted, it also steps up your metabolic rate, often for up to several hours after an activity.

If you're following your Diet Type, a brisk, deep-breathing forty-five minute walk a day or its equivalent* can subtract an extra 20 pounds a year. One study found that people who exercised vigorously four or five times a week lost weight at a safe, steady pace—and three times faster than those who worked out three times a week (less than this has virtually no effect). Such aerobic, muscle-powering exercise has just the opposite impact of frequent dieting. By reshaping and firming your body, it can reduce your measurements by one or two clothing sizes and make you look leaner even if you don't lose a pound of scale weight.† Keeping vigorously active is especially crucial as you age, since the body loses lean muscle and replaces it with fat more readily later in life.

---

* Swimming, cycling, brisk walking, jogging or a good running tennis game for twenty to thirty minutes; and cross-country skiing or rope-jumping for ten to twelve minutes are also good alternatives.

† Actually, lean muscle weighs more than fat, so your scale weight may not necessarily drop dramatically.

BEYOND THE SCALE

What counts above all is the percentage of fat on your body, not the numbers on your bathroom scale. It's possible to have a normal weight according to standard tables, yet still be "overfat." Among the best methods for gauging body fat are underwater weighing, skinfold tests and a new painless device called the body composition analysis machine. It will tell you how much of your weight is bone, water, organs and muscle, and how much is actually fat. During his prime, football star Mark Gastineau's 260-pound, 6-foot frame was only 6% fat! Despite the hefty number on his scale, he did not have a weight problem.

Typically, women of normal weight should have about 20 to 30 percent body fat, and men, about 12 to 21 percent. Remember, keeping your diet low in fats will guarantee that little, if any, of what you eat turns into extra pounds of fat on your body.

IS YOUR THYROID TO BLAME?

Probably not. Many of the chronically overweight have attributed their problem to a sluggish thyroid, but this belief is vastly oversimplified and has led some to view thyroid medication as a panacea. In fact, people who develop hypothyroidism, or an underactive thyroid, do not necessarily become fat. Their body's metabolic rate drops somewhat and they become less physically active, but they are not likely to eat enough to gain a significant amount of weight.

If tests show you are not making enough thyroxine, supplements can help turn you from torpid to energetic and raise your metabolic rate—both important for lasting weight loss. However, excessive or unnecessary thyroid medication for any length of time can result in rapid or irregular heartbeat, nervousness, insomnia, muscle weakness and bone loss. It can also be psychologically addicting, leading you to require substantial amounts indefinitely to "control" your weight.

On the other hand, while it may not have a direct impact on body weight, even a mildly malfunctioning thyroid can trigger a range of debilitating symptoms, including fatigue, malaise, difficulty in breathing, swollen feet, depression and headaches. Another subtle side effect is increased susceptibility to infection, since an underactive thyroid causes low immunity. The thyroid has even been linked recently with premenstrual syndrome, or PMS. A study of thirty-one women with premenstrual complaints showed that all of them improved when given low doses of thyroxine. Any one of these problems could interfere with efforts to lose weight.

Sometimes it's possible to correct a thyroid imbalance simply by compensating for vitamin and mineral deficiencies with moderate doses of iodine or the amino acid tyrosine, a raw material for thyroid hormone, along with B vitamins, zinc and copper. However, thyroid extract is necessary in some cases. Many patients are concerned that supplements will make their thyroid gland "lazy," so that it stops producing any hormone at all. But for those truly in need, thyroid medication is a gentle, temporary crutch that can give an overstressed gland a holiday. Often that holiday helps the organ heal, so it can resume function beautifully on its own.

BEYOND BIOLOGY

For many people, biology is largely beside the point. Their relationship to food is primarily *emotional*, as are their reasons for overeating. Like drugs or alcohol, a meal may represent an escape from loneliness, anxiety, depression, sexual conflict or job stress. If the underlying source of trouble is not resolved, a serious weight problem could result. Perhaps early in life such individuals learned from their parents or from family eating patterns that food represented love, affection, nurturing—the panacea for all ills. Or maybe they weren't loved enough and turned to food for emotional support. Popular diet and fitness authority Richard Simmons recalls that while growing up, he often consoled himself with large amounts of sweets because he thought his parents loved his older brother more. Eating is also associated with strongly positive emotions and occasions—holidays, celebrations, weddings, family outings, barbecues. It's socially sanctioned (and also legal!), something we may do without restraint when we're feeling wonderful, terrible or otherwise in need of an emotional fix.

An array of environmental cues, or outside influences, can induce us to eat for reasons other than hunger, and they can be far more persuasive than the inner signals that tell us when we're full. Overweight people are believed to be more susceptible than usual to external pressures and enticements, and less in touch with their own internal cues. In other words, they have trouble distinguishing between real hunger and just plain temptation. For example, some may be especially sensitive to the sight, smell and taste of food. Others may feel an overwhelming urge to eat if they merely *think* about a meal. One of my patients had an irresistible craving whenever she passed a certain pizza shop on her way home. Another patient claimed that the sound of his office clock striking noon was enough to send him into a "frenzy" for food.

If you have something of a herd instinct, it may be difficult to stay away from food when family or friends are indulging. Whether it's boredom, habit, social pressures, mental or visual stimuli or relief from unpleasant emotions, find out what environmental "green lights" are signaling you to eat. Realize that you can respond to any of these signals in ways other than eating. The simple necessity—and pleasure—of eating often gets obscured by all the extraneous and unhealthy reasons for it. The solution is for you—on your own, in a support group or with professional help—to identify these situations and then either avoid them or substitute ways of dealing with them that won't compromise your health.

FOR *ALL* DIETERS: A MATTER OF FAT

Besides proving that edible fat turns easily into body fat, scientists have made other key discoveries about this familiar diet taboo. Most of us are aware that saturated fats are harmful to health, but few suspect how widespread they are in our diets. The obvious ones are found in most foods of animal origin, such as beef, pork, lamb and whole dairy products. Trimming the fat off a steak, however, or simply cutting down on butter and sour cream may be far from enough. If you eat any processed foods at all, be aware that vast numbers of them contain hydrogenated or partially hydrogenated oils, which, although unsaturated, are chemically similar to saturated fats and act the same way in our body, increasing our risk of heart disease. In fact, they are among the most frequently used ingredients in foods, and can be found in margarine, breads, cakes and cake mixes, pies, cookies, muffin mixes, crackers, boxed snacks, commercial peanut butter, granola bars, some presweetened and honeyed breakfast cereals, ice cream cones, packaged rice and stuffing mixes, prepared bread crumbs, croutons and some frozen foods, among many others. Likewise, watch out for any label boasting, "made with 100% pure vegetable shortening," for the two most commonly used vegetable oils—coconut and palm kernel—are more saturated than beef fat!

Unfortunately, polyunsaturated oils, widely touted as a safe alternative for diet-minded eaters, may be just as detrimental to health. While they have been duly credited with lowering blood cholesterol, they are indiscriminate, since they reduce the beneficial as well as the harmful cholesterol (see below). Like saturated fats, they promote the clumping of red blood cells and platelets that can lead to arterial blockage. What's more, they may raise the risk of developing cancer. In repeated studies, they have been associated with a higher incidence of tumors in laboratory animals. Apparently, they oxidize (break down chemically) and become rancid within the body quite easily, releasing destructive molecular particles called free radicals. As their name suggests, the latter roam carelessly among cells, disrupting their functions and doing damage to both their internal genetic code and outer membranes, making them more vulnerable to carcinogens.

What about cholesterol? While this special type of fat is essential to nerves, cell membranes, vital organs (including the brain) and many hormones, the body has no dietary need for it, because the liver manufactures enough on its own. The often mentioned distinction between "good" and "bad" cholesterol refers to the fatty proteins (lipoproteins) that attach themselves to cholesterol and carry it through the bloodstream. The "good" kind—HDLs, or high-density lipoprotens—helps convey cholesterol out of the body via the liver. The "bad" LDLs and VLDLs (low-density and very-low-density lipoproteins) escort cholesterol to the body's tissues and often deposit it on arterial walls.

Most people are believed to have a homeostatic, or self-balancing, capacity that allows them to adapt to any short-term cholesterol challenge. A number of studies have shown that giving several eggs a day to people who have normal blood-cholesterol levels and otherwise sensible low-fat diets leaves their cholesterol profiles virtually unchanged. Their bodies respond by reducing the amount of cholesterol they absorb from foods or synthesize on their own. In an experiment conducted by research dietitian Jacqueline Edington at the Radcliffe Infirmary in Oxford, England, 168 subjects were given two eggs a week for eight weeks and then seven eggs a week for the same amount of time. Concurrently, they followed a relatively low-fat diet, ate more fiber and reduced their intake of saturated fats. No one showed any rise in serum cholesterol. (However, don't interpret this finding as a license to overeat eggs. One recent experiment did show that too many added to the diet may produce more of a certain lipoprotein that *acts* just like LDLs and may do even more damage.)

A recent University of Arizona report finds that about two-thirds of the population need not worry unduly about cholesterol intake. Our liver and cells make all the cholesterol we need, so it is *not* a required nutrient. Since we use a relatively small amount for essential functions like the synthesis of sex hormones and fat-digesting bile acids, the body normally excretes any excess and cuts down on the amount it produces. However, some people seem to be "wired" genetically to produce more cholesterol than others, regardless of their eating habits. In fact, about one-quarter to one-third of the population may be unable to metabolize or regulate cholesterol properly, or to adapt well to any outside increase, and the surplus builds up gradually in body tissues, heightening the risk of cardiovascular disease.

In some cases, the people who are oversensitive to dietary cholesterol have a condition known as hypercholesterolemia, which often runs in families. If you have such a history, you should be extra careful about your intake of both saturated fats and cholesterol, especially the former. This is because most LDL-type cholesterol in the body—the kind that "sticks"—results from an excess of saturated fat, *not* cholesterol itself. Saturated fats are the raw material from which cholesterol is made and are the critical factor when it comes to raising blood levels of cholesterol. Sure enough, serum cholesterol can be *lowered* by substantially reducing dietary fat. In Ms. Edington's study, for example, participants showed a marked drop in cholesterol when they initially switched to a low-fat diet.

However, two types of fat are friendly to the beneficial HDL cholesterol and so should be part of any diet. These are the monounsaturated oils—principally olive, avocado, soy and canola (rapeseed) oil—which lower the undesirable LDLs while preserving or even raising the HDLs, and fatty fish oils, with their own unique class of polyunsaturates. These oils offer a number of benefits, including protection against heart and coronary artery disease, hypertension, inflammatory disorders such as rheumatoid arthritis, and even certain forms of cancer. The best news for fat-wary dieters is that small amounts of both monounsaturates and fish oils are enough to deliver these advantages.

How Low Should Cholesterol Be?

Back in the 1960s, the relationship between cholesterol and heart disease started to become evident, but scientific journals kept publishing disclaimer editorials with titles like "The Diet/Heart Disease Connection: A Premature Inference?" In their plodding conservatism, many mainstream nutritionists ignored the possible benefits that sweeping dietary recommendations for lowering saturated-fat and cholesterol intake could have on the health of the American populace.

Now, after twenty-odd years of acrimonious debate, these entrenched academics have conceded that lowering cholesterol intake should be a national dietary priority. Recently the American Heart Association further revised its ideal cholesterol recommendations *downward*, suggesting that cholesterol for middle-aged patients register at maximum in the low 200s. Some contend that the numbers should be even lower. These advocates point out that when cholesterol reaches a level of 160 or less in a given population, the incidence of heart disease becomes virtually nil.

Can cholesterol be *too* low? Some studies show that people with low cholesterol—140 or less—tend to have a higher incidence of immune-deficiency disease, such as cancer, AIDS and other viral infections. I often notice this in my own patients. But the explanation is not that they are obtaining too little cholesterol from their diets. Rather, their low reading is a reflection of some metabolic change that occurs when the immune system is weakened. Experiments have shown that cancerous cells may feed off the body's cholesterol, lowering it to subnormal levels. My recommendation to patients with lowered immunity is not to eat fatty foods to raise their cholesterol but rather to adopt a natural high-fiber, predominantly vegetarian diet to enhance their immune systems.

What role does diet play in regulating cholesterol? Where do hereditary factors enter in? This varies. Because of their genetic makeup some people can lower their cholesterol only minimally by altering their diets. I recall the recent case of a superbly trained woman athlete, following a strict Pritikin Diet, who came to my office with a cholesterol level of nearly 400. Her brothers had all died of heart attacks in their thirties. She was suffering from a genetic defect in her ability to eliminate excess cholesterol, and dietary changes alone did not reduce her blood cholesterol levels beyond a certain point. On the other hand, the *vast majority* of my patients can reduce theirs by as much as 100 points in as short a time as six to eight week through aggressive dietary manipulation.

A recent study completed in the South, called "The Bogalusa Heart Study," shows that dietary intervention to prevent heart disease should begin early. Autopsy specimens of male teenage victims of violent death due to car accident, stabbing or gunshot wounds have revealed that many of them had well-advanced narrowing of the arteries due to cholesterol plaques. The extent of the damage was correlated with the amount of fat consumed and with cigarette smoking, even at an early age. The recommendation now is that even children be screened for tendency toward high cholesterol, particularly if a parent has developed heart disease before the age of sixty.

As for the right diet strategy, fiber itself appears to be beneficial in preventing the absorption of cholesterol and in accelerating its excretion from the body. However, the most valuable kind of fiber is not the coarse bran which many of us have dutifully poured on our morning cereals, but rather the soft, soluble fiber best exemplified by oat bran, beans and certain vegetables and fruits, such as pectin-rich carrots and apples. Studies have shown that the addition of oat bran and beans even to a diet high in cholesterol can help lower blood levels of cholesterol significantly. Such findings will

NO MORE CHOLESTEROL CONTROVERSY

In the '70s, when I was in medical school, we were in the midst of the "cholesterol controversy." I remember engaging in heated debates with some of my conservative professors about the extent to which fat-lowering recommendations should be made for the general population. "It is premature," they used to say in the measured tones of scientific orthodoxy, "to make recommendations to all patients regarding their animal-fat and cholesterol intake. We just don't know yet if it has a direct bearing on heart disease!"

These days, I feel vindicated. No longer is it the era of the "cholesterol controversy"; we are now firmly in the age of the "cholesterol connection." No less an authority than the prestigious National Institutes of Health (NIH) has recently introduced guidelines that would have been considered radical just five or ten years ago. While patients with cholesterol levels of less than 200 need no specific therapy, those with levels of only 200 to 240 are at "moderate risk" for heart disease and should lower saturated-fat and cholesterol intake as well as maintain ideal weight. People with cholesterol greater than 240 (a number until recently viewed with complacency by most doctors) are now considered to be at high risk and should modify their diets even more stringently.

The results can be striking. A recent National Heart, Lung and Blood Institute collaborative study estimates that for each 1 percent reduction in blood cholesterol there is an approximate 2 percent reduction in the incidence of coronary heart disease!

be discussed in greater detail in the chapter on the High-Fiber/Super Grain Diet.

Surprisingly, certain proteins, regardless of their cholesterol or fat content, have an impact on serum cholesterol. Most people believe that by eating low-fat cottage cheese and skim milk they are exempt from the cholesterol-raising properties of dairy foods. But it has been found that casein, the chief protein in all milk products, is capable of boosting cholesterol whether or not it keeps the company of saturated fat or cholesterol. On the other hand, consuming soy protein has a cholesterol-*lowering* effect. The kind of meat you eat can be crucial, too. A recent analysis of the "caveman diet" shows that although prehistoric man ate a fair amount of meat, it was far lower in saturated fat and cholesterol than what supermarkets supply today. Wild game meat is much higher in protective Omega-3 fatty acids as well as mono- and polyunsaturates than its "civilized" counterpart. More revelations about the effects of different kinds of proteins will be discussed in the chapter on the Modified Protein-Plus Diet.

EXERCISE VS. CHOLESTEROL

For most people, exercise reinforces the effects of a sensible diet since it elevates levels of HDL cholesterol. It is not unusual for me to see well-trained athletes—swimmers, cyclists, runners—in my office with HDL readings ranging as high as 90, 100 or 110. Jogging for as little as nine miles a week is beneficial. And one study showed increased HDL levels in mail carriers who walked five miles a day.

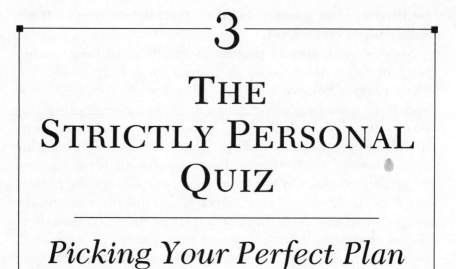

3

THE STRICTLY PERSONAL QUIZ

Picking Your Perfect Plan

Diet books typically assume a one-eating-plan-fits-all approach, prescribing the same how-tos and promising identical results to everyone regardless of lifestyle, medical status or need. In effect, such books suggest that people in quest of nutritional well-being and slimmer bodies all eat, think and act alike. They do not consider the possibility that a diet can succeed only if it conforms to your personal profile and is essentially made to order.

The following questionnaire, divided into four sections, will help you identify your eating attitudes, preferences, habits and beliefs as well as your diet and medical history to discover the best Diet Type for you. Please complete each question by circling the appropriate letter, then transfer your answers to the score sheet at the end of the questionnaire. By tallying your score for each of the Diet Types listed in this book, you will increase your chances of finding a safe, successful regimen that can serve you for life. Instructions for scoring your diet-type responses will be given on page 53. Meanwhile, relax and enjoy the test—and remember, while we're not grading you, *be as honest as you can.*

Diet Questionnaire

SECTION I: Behavior and Preferences

In this section, we'll evaluate the kind of individual you are, as well as your eating, shopping and dining behavior and attitudes. Answer "true" (T) or "false" (F).

1. I rarely have the time to buy fresh food.   **T**   **F**

2. I am a student or live in a residential situation where food is provided.   **T**   **F**

3. I almost invariably eat out.   **T**   **F**

4. I'm appalled by the standard American diet.   **T**   **F**

5. I'm convinced that "real" men and women don't eat health food!   **T**   **F**

6. I find health food boring.   **T**   **F**

7. For me, a healthy diet is a primary goal, and if weight loss "just happens," so much the better.   **T**   **F**

8. For me, weight loss is a primary goal, even if the foods I eat are not the healthiest.   **T**   **F**

9. I have too little time to cook or eat anything but "convenience" foods.   **T**   **F**

10. I enjoy cooking and following new recipes.   **T**   **F**

11. I am required by my work to have frequent business meals in "mainstream" restaurants.　　T　F

12. Food restrictions would make me feel weird or left out in the company of others.　　T　F

13. My spouse/children/parents/roommate(s) make it hard for me to radically change my diet.　　T　F

14. In my community, health food restaurants are easy to find.　　T　F

15. I travel a lot to places where health food is unavailable or inaccessible.　　T　F

16. I consider myself exotic and experimental when it comes to making food choices.　　T　F

17. I like to shop in health-food stores.　　T　F

18. In my community, health-food stores are relatively accessible.　　T　F

19. I would hate to be bothered with measuring or weighing portions.　　T　F

20. I need food that "sticks to my ribs"; eating in a Chinese restaurant leaves me hungry just a few hours after.　　T　F

21. I need a hearty breakfast every morning or I feel weak and tired.　　T　F

22. After most meals I feel heavy and weighted down.　　T　F

23. The idea of rotating my foods from one day to another seems difficult or impossible.　　T　F

24. I would enjoy and be comfortable with eating just fruit for breakfast.　　T　F

25. I believe the ideal diet would be mostly vegetarian.   **T**   **F**

26. I feel "spacy" and/or tired within minutes after eating.   **T**   **F**

27. I have difficulty going for long periods without eating.   **T**   **F**

28. I require specific instructions as to how much to eat at each mealtime.   **T**   **F**

29. I tend to binge and overeat, whether it's "junk" or the healthiest possible food.   **T**   **F**

30. I tend to get stuck on a single food or a few perennial favorites.   **T**   **F**

31. I crave fruits, juices and sweets.   **T**   **F**

32. I crave cheese, milk, cream and butter.   **T**   **F**

33. I constantly crave pasta, potatoes and bread.   **T**   **F**

34. I have lots of gas and bloating when eating a vegetarian diet heavy in beans and whole grains.   **T**   **F**

35. I enjoy shopping for food.   **T**   **F**

36. I insist on buying fresh produce and other ingredients.   **T**   **F**

37. I don't know what I'd do without canned and frozen foods.   **T**   **F**

38. Counting calories drives me crazy.   **T**   **F**

39. At work (home) I'm near a lot of fast-food restaurants and I depend on them a lot.   **T**   **F**

40. I eat primarily for enjoyment; being able to eat whatever I like is an important part of my well-being and health.   **T**   **F**

41. If I miss a meal, I feel uncomfortable (dizzy, fatigued, headachy, drowsy or irritable).　　T　F

42. I get relief from these discomforts if I eat.　　T　F

43. I make sure that I have my favorite foods in the house every day.　　T　F

44. I think counting calories is an effective way to lose weight.　　T　F

45. I tend to eat all day long; I'm always munching, nibbling or snacking on something.　　T　F

46. I enjoy trying new, exotic cuisines and dishes in restaurants and/or experimenting with new ways of cooking.　　T　F

47. I can't live without meat.　　T　F

48. I'm a real salad gourmet.　　T　F

49. I'm a light eater, especially in the summer.　　T　F

50. I must have protein at every meal or else I walk away feeling hungry.　　T　F

51. I like eating three square meals a day.　　T　F

52. I'm so busy I usually eat my meals on the run.　　T　F

53. I hate to cook or shop for food, and am a restaurant junkie.　　T　F

54. I generally prefer to eat several smaller meals throughout the day.　　T　F

55. There's nothing like the sight/smell of a steak or hamburger sizzling on the grill.　　T　F

56. Meat should be part of a good, satisfying, balanced meal.　　T　F

57. Whenever I'm abroad, I get homesick for real American food.   **T**   **F**

58. I consider diet my first line of defense against cancer and heart disease.   **T**   **F**

59. I like ritual and am drawn to diets that are based on some form of philosophy or tradition.   **T**   **F**

60. I would rather be told what and when to eat than be left with too many choices.   **T**   **F**

61. I have the same foods day in and day out.   **T**   **F**

62. I feel there are some foods that I just couldn't live without.   **T**   **F**

63. I would find it difficult to make it through the day without my typical morning or mid-afternoon snack consisting of a particular food that I crave at those times.   **T**   **F**

64. I have a hard time falling asleep without that certain special bedtime food.   **T**   **F**

SECTION II: Foods

In this section, we'll determine which basic categories of foods you prefer.

	Like	Am indifferent to	Dislike
65. Whole-grain breads and cereals (bulgur, pearl barley, brown rice, rolled oats, kasha)	A	B	C
66. "Good old" American cuisine	A	B	C
67. Dairy foods (cheese, milk, yogurt, butter)	A	B	C

	Like	Am indifferent to	Dislike
68. Vegetable protein (tofu, beans, miso, tempeh, soy milk)	A	B	C
69. Fresh fruits, raw vegetables, salads, sprouts, vegetable and fruit juices.	A	B	C
70. Canned, frozen, "convenience" foods	A	B	C
71. Oriental, Middle Eastern and/or Italian cuisine	A	B	C
72. Red meat (beef, pork, lamb, veal, organ meat)	A	B	C
73. Low-calorie "diet desserts," e.g., Weight Watchers products	A	B	C

SECTION III: Dieting History

In this section, we'll examine your reactions to some of the popular diets.

	Like or found helpful	Have no opinion about or don't know	Disliked or did not find helpful
74. Weight Watchers, Diet Center programs	A	B	C
75. Macrobiotics	A	B	C
76. Dr. Atkins'/Stillman/ Scarsdale diets (high protein)	A	B	C
77. *Fit for Life* or Natural Hygiene (raw vegetables and fruits)	A	B	C

	Like or found helpful	Have no opinion about or don't know	Disliked or did not find helpful
78. Dr. Berger's Immune Power Diet (antiallergy)	A	B	C
79. Pritikin Program, F-Plan, McDougall Plan (high fiber)	A	B	C
80. The Anti-Candida Diet, *The Yeast Connection* (antiallergy)	A	B	C
81. Ovo-lacto-vegetarian Diet (moderate eggs, dairy)	A	B	C

SECTION IV: Medical History

In this final and most important section, we'll determine which diet is healthiest for you. Answer "yes" (Y) or "no" (N).

Family History:

82. Do two or more of your parents or siblings suffer from adult-onset diabetes?   Y N

83. Do two or more of your parents, siblings or children suffer from debilitating allergies (chronic nasal congestion, asthma, eczema or hives)?   Y N

84. Do you have one or more parents, siblings or children who have suffered from colon cancer?   Y N

85. Do you have one or more parents or siblings who suffered from heart disease (heart attack or angina) before the age of sixty?   Y N

86. (women only) Do you have a mother, sister, grandmother or daughter who has had breast cancer?   Y N

Personal History:

87. Do you have a history of kidney disease, or have you been told by a physician of reduced kidney function? Y N

88. Do you have a tendency toward anemia or a history of iron or vitamin B-12 deficiency? Y N

89. Do you have rheumatoid arthritis? Y N

90. Do you have gallstones (not surgically removed)? Y N

91. Have you had kidney stones? Y N

92. Do you have a history of gout? Y N

93. Are you chronically constipated and/or do you have painful hemorrhoids? Y N

94. Have you been diagnosed as allergic to foods or candida (yeast)? Y N

95. (women only) Do you have extremely painful periods or the condition of endometriosis? Y N

96. Have you ever been diagnosed as having hypoglycemia (low blood sugar)? Y N

97. Have you ever been diagnosed as having cancer of the breast, colon, rectum, uterus, ovary or prostate? Y N

98. Have you been told you have diverticulosis/diverticulitis (intestinal outpocketings with a tendency to become infected)? Y N

99. Have you been told you have high cholesterol or triglycerides (or is your fasting serum cholesterol greater than 200 mg/dl and/or your fasting serum triglycerides greater than 160 mg/dl)? Y N

100. Is your fasting serum cholesterol greater than 240 mg, or are your fasting serum triglycerides greater than 250?*   Y   N

101. If you know your serum *HDL* cholesterol as well as your *total* cholesterol, compute your cholesterol/HDL ratio by dividing total cholesterol by HDL. Is your cholesterol/HDL ratio greater than 5?*   Y   N

102. Do you have severe emphysema or restrictive lung disease?   Y   N

103. Do you have a history of diabetes?   Y   N

104. Do you have a history of allergies (chronic nasal congestion, asthma, eczema or hives)?   Y   N

105. Do you have a history of heart attack, angina, stroke or claudication (pain in legs due to arteriosclerosis)?   Y   N

106. Do you have a history of high blood pressure?   Y   N

107. Are your teeth bad, or do you have difficulty chewing?   Y   N

108. Do you tend to have facial puffiness, bags under the eyes or water retention?   Y   N

SCORE SHEET

Now that you have completed the diet questionnaire, transfer your answers to the following score sheet. This sheet will help translate your responses into specific diet recommendations. Each of your answers has been assigned a point

*See "Testing for Cholesterol: What the Numbers Mean" at the end of this chapter.

value corresponding to each of the five basic Diet Types outlined in this book.

For example, if you answered "true" on question 1, circle the letter T opposite question 1 on the score sheet, then follow the arrow to the group of numbers on the right and circle them, as follows:

	A	B	C	D	E
1. (T) ────────────────→	(1	2	2	0	3)
F ────────────────→	0	0	0	0	0

Similarly, if you answered "false," you would follow the arrow from F to the group of numbers at right.

SECTION I

	A	B	C	D	E			A	B	C	D	E
1. T →	1	2	2	0	3		9. T →	0	0	0	0	3
F →	2	0	0	3	0		F →	0	0	0	0	0
2. T →	0	2	1	1	3		10. T →	3	1	2	3	1
F →	0	0	0	0	0		F →	0	2	1	0	3
3. T →	0	2	1	0	3		11. T →	0	2	1	0	3
F →	0	0	0	0	0		F →	0	0	0	0	0
4. T →	3	0	1	3	0		12. T →	0	2	1	0	3
F →	0	3	0	0	3		F →	0	0	0	0	0
5. T →	0	3	0	0	3		13. T →	0	2	1	0	3
F →	3	1	1	3	0		F →	0	0	0	0	0
6. T →	0	3	0	0	3		14. T →	3	0	0	3	0
F →	3	1	1	3	0		F →	0	2	1	0	3
7. T →	3	0	1	3	0		15. T →	0	2	1	0	3
F →	0	3	1	0	3		F →	0	0	0	0	0
8. T →	0	2	0	0	3		16. T →	3	0	0	3	0
F →	3	1	0	3	0		F →	0	3	2	0	3

		A	B	C	D	E
17.	T →	3	0	0	3	0
	F →	0	3	3	0	3
18.	T →	3	0	0	3	0
	F →	0	3	3	0	3
19.	T →	3	3	3	3	0
	F →	0	0	0	0	3
20.	T →	0	3	2	0	2
	F →	3	0	1	3	1
21.	T →	3	3	3	0	3
	F →	0	0	0	3	0
22.	T →	2	0	1	3	1
	F →	0	0	0	0	0
23.	T →	3	3	0	3	3
	F →	0	0	3	0	0
24.	T →	0	0	0	3	0
	F →	3	3	3	0	3
25.	T →	3	0	0	3	0
	F →	0	3	3	0	3
26.	T →	3	3	3	0	0
	F →	0	0	0	0	0
27.	T →	3	4	0	0	0
	F →	0	0	0	0	0
28.	T →	0	0	0	0	3
	F →	0	0	0	0	0
29.	T →	0	0	0	0	3
	F →	0	0	0	0	0
30.	T →	0	0	5	0	0
	F →	0	0	0	0	0
31.	T →	3	3	0	0	0
	F →	0	0	0	0	0

		A	B	C	D	E
32.	T →	3	0	3	3	0
	F →	0	0	0	0	0
33.	T →	0	3	3	0	0
	F →	0	0	0	0	0
34.	T →	0	3	2	1	2
	F →	2	0	0	2	0
35.	T →	3	1	3	3	1
	F →	0	3	0	0	3
36.	T →	3	0	1	3	0
	F →	0	3	1	0	3
37.	T →	0	0	0	0	3
	F →	3	1	1	3	0
38.	T →	3	3	3	3	0
	F →	0	0	0	0	3
39.	T →	0	0	0	0	3
	F →	0	0	0	0	0
40.	T →	0	0	0	0	3
	F →	0	0	0	0	0
41.	T →	2	0	3	2	1
	F →	0	0	0	0	0
42.	T →	2	0	3	2	1
	F →	0	0	0	0	0
43.	T →	0	0	3	0	0
	F →	0	0	0	0	0
44.	T →	0	0	0	0	3
	F →	3	2	2	3	0
45.	T →	0	0	0	3	0
	F →	0	0	0	0	0
46.	T →	3	0	0	3	0
	F →	0	0	0	0	3

	A	B	C	D	E			A	B	C	D	E
47. T →	0	3	1	0	2		56. T →	0	3	1	0	2
F →	3	0	1	3	1		F →	3	0	1	3	1
48. T →	2	0	0	3	0		57. T →	0	1	1	0	3
F →	0	3	0	0	2		F →	2	1	1	2	0
49. T →	1	0	0	3	0		58. T →	3	0	0	3	0
F →	1	2	2	0	2		F →	0	3	3	0	3
50. T →	1	3	1	0	2		59. T →	3	1	3	3	0
F →	2	0	0	3	0		F →	0	1	0	0	3
51. T →	2	2	2	0	2		60. T →	1	1	3	1	0
F →	0	0	0	2	0		F →	1	1	0	1	3
52. T →	0	0	0	0	3		61. T →	0	0	3	0	0
F →	0	0	0	0	0		F →	0	0	0	0	0
53. T →	0	2	0	0	3		62. T →	0	0	3	0	0
F →	0	0	0	0	0		F →	0	0	0	0	0
54. T →	0	0	0	2	0		63. T →	0	0	3	0	0
F →	0	0	0	0	0		F →	0	0	0	0	0
55. T →	0	3	1	0	2		64. T →	0	0	3	0	0
F →	3	0	1	3	1		F →	0	0	0	0	0

SECTION II

	A	B	C	D	E			A	B	C	D	E
65. A →	3	0	0	3	0		68. A →	3	0	0	3	0
B →	0	0	0	0	0		B →	0	0	0	0	0
C →	0	3	3	0	3		C →	0	3	0	0	3
66. A →	0	3	1	0	3		69. A →	2	0	1	3	1
B →	0	0	0	0	0		B →	0	0	0	0	0
C →	3	0	1	3	0		C →	1	3	2	0	2
67. A →	0	3	3	0	3		70. A →	0	0	0	0	3
B →	0	0	0	0	0		B →	0	0	0	0	0
C →	3	0	1	3	0		C →	3	3	3	3	0

	A	B	C	D	E			A	B	C	D	E
71. A→	3	0	0	2	0		73. A→	0	0	0	0	3
B→	0	0	0	0	0		B→	0	0	0	0	0
C→	0	3	3	1	3		C→	3	3	3	3	0
72. A→	0	3	3	0	3							
B→	0	0	0	0	0							
C→	3	0	0	3	0							

SECTION III

	A	B	C	D	E			A	B	C	D	E
74. A→	0	0	0	0	3		78. A→	0	0	3	0	0
B→	0	0	0	0	0		B→	0	0	0	0	0
C→	3	3	3	3	0		C→	3	3	0	3	3
75. A→	3	0	0	2	0		79. A→	3	0	0	2	0
B→	0	0	0	0	0		B→	0	0	0	0	0
C→	0	3	3	1	3		C→	0	3	3	1	3
76. A→	0	3	1	0	2		80. A→	1	1	3	0	0
B→	0	0	0	0	0		B→	0	0	0	0	0
C→	3	0	1	3	0		C→	3	1	0	3	3
77. A→	1	0	0	3	0		81. A→	3	0	0	3	0
B→	0	0	0	0	0		B→	0	0	0	0	0
C→	1	3	1	0	3		C→	0	3	3	0	3

SECTION IV

	A	B	C	D	E			A	B	C	D	E
82. Y→	2	0	1	2	0		85. Y→	3	0	0	3	0
N→	0	0	0	0	0		N→	0	0	0	0	0
83. Y→	0	1	3	1	0		86. Y	3	0	0	3	0
N→	0	0	0	0	0		N→	0	0	0	0	0
84. Y→	3	0	0	3	0		87. Y→	3	3	0	-3	0
N→	0	0	0	0	0		N→	0	0	0	0	0

		A	B	C	D	E
88.	Y →	0	0	1	0	1
	N →	0	0	0	0	0
89.	Y →	3	0	3	3	0
	N →	0	0	0	0	0
90.	Y →	3	0	0	3	0
	N →	0	0	0	0	0
91.	Y →	3	0	0	2	0
	N →	0	0	0	0	0
92.	Y →	3	−3	0	3	0
	N →	0	0	0	0	0
93.	Y →	3	0	0	3	0
	N	0	0	0	0	0
94.	Y →	0	0	5	0	0
	N →	0	0	0	0	0
95.	Y →	3	0	0	3	0
	N →	0	0	0	0	0
96.	Y →	3	3	0	0	0
	N →	0	0	0	0	0
97.	Y →	3	0	0	3	0
	N →	0	0	0	0	0
98.	Y →	3	0	0	3	0
	N →	0	0	0	0	0

		A	B	C	D	E
99.	Y →	3	−5	0	3	0
	N →	0	0	0	0	0
100.	Y →	3	0	0	3	0
	N →	0	0	0	0	0
101.	Y →	3	−5	0	3	0
	N →	0	0	0	0	0
102.	Y →	0	3	0	0	0
	N →	0	0	0	0	0
103.	Y →	3	0	1	3	0
	N →	0	0	0	0	0
104.	Y →	0	1	5	1	0
	N →	0	0	0	0	0
105.	Y →	3	−5	0	3	0
	N →	0	0	0	0	0
106.	Y →	3	0	0	3	0
	N →	0	0	0	0	0
107.	Y →	0	3	3	0	3
	N →	0	0	0	0	0
108.	Y →	0	0	3	0	0
	N →	0	0	0	0	0

DECIDING YOUR DIET-TYPE

After all the number groups next to your answers have been circled, vertically scan each column of numbers and add them. You may wish to use a calculator for this. Come up with a cumulative point total **for each of columns A through E.**

Example:

ADD THE POINT SCORES IN EACH COLUMN

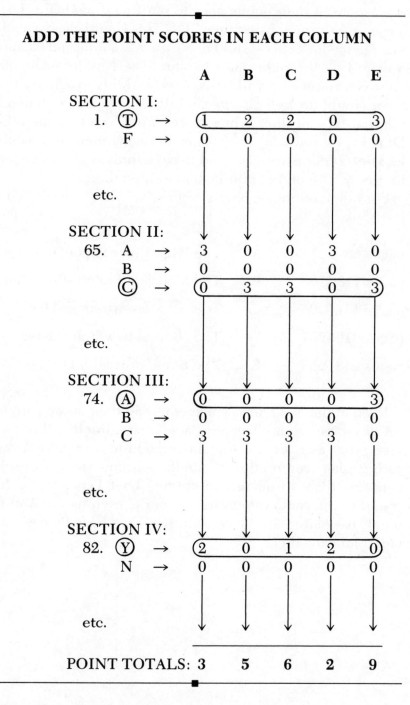

	A	B	C	D	E
SECTION I:					
1. Ⓣ →	1	2	2	0	3
F →	0	0	0	0	0
etc.					
SECTION II:					
65. A →	3	0	0	3	0
B →	0	0	0	0	0
Ⓒ →	0	3	3	0	3
etc.					
SECTION III:					
74. Ⓐ →	0	0	0	0	3
B →	0	0	0	0	0
C →	3	3	3	3	0
etc.					
SECTION IV:					
82. Ⓨ →	2	0	1	2	0
N →	0	0	0	0	0
etc.					
POINT TOTALS:	3	5	6	2	9

For the person filling out this hypothetical partial quiz, the high score of nine points goes to the Bored of Health Diet-Type, represented by column "E." This would clearly be the first choice for a successful Diet-Type match-up, and Chapter 8 would be the right place to start. The No-More-Allergies Diet is a runner-up with six points, and this imaginary test-taker would do well also to carefully study Chapter 6 detailing that type of diet. While scores were lower on the other Diet Types, reducing the chance for using them, our would-be Diet Typer is well advised to page through those sections for the wealth of diet information located there.

For quick reference here's where each diet is described in the book:

pages 68–117	A	The High Fiber/Super Grain Diet
pages 118–166	B	The Modified Protein-Plus Diet
pages 167–209	C	The No-More-Allergies Diet
pages 210–257	D	The Natural Raw Foods Diet
pages 258–288	E	The Bored of Health Diet

Each of the five Diet-Type menus and their accompanying set of recipes should serve as a general guideline. Follow a given diet as is or use it as inspiration to design your own eating plan, conforming to similar portion sizes. Consider choosing dishes from any of the five Diet Types that correspond to the same categories in your chosen menu. And for quick, easy alternatives, consult the "Five Easy Pieces" provided for each diet.

TESTING FOR CHOLESTEROL:
WHAT THE NUMBERS MEAN

A healthy, slim thirty-two-year-old recently found out from a routine blood test that his cholesterol is 220. His doctor told him that this was "okay," without offering any further explanation. However, the patient remains troubled, since he has heard some physicians recommend a cholesterol of less than 200. He is also aware that one component of total cholesterol is desirable, and would like to know how much of his 220 falls in this category.

As for the numbers and their significance, recognize that cholesterol levels may fluctuate widely from lab to lab, and even from day to day in the same individual. Test results vary depending on the time of day blood is drawn and whether the patient is lying down or sitting. Since the margin for error is so great, any questionable cholesterol values warrant a second test.

The amount of HDL cholesterol, or high-density lipoproteins, is a very important index of cardiovascular risk and should always be measured to complete your cholesterol profile. This special type of fatty particle helps filter excess cholesterol from the blood and thus prevent it from collecting on artery walls; the presence of HDLs in sufficient quantities has been associated with lowered risk of heart attack and stroke. A total cholesterol reading of 220 may be good or bad news, depending on your HDL level. In most men, the average HDL figure is about 45, and in women, who are at lower risk of heart disease, it is about 50. A number of less than 35 should cause you to rethink your diet (unless your total cholesterol is safely below the 180–200 range), while an index

(Continued)

(Continued)

higher than 55 suggests that your eating habits may be beyond reproach!

If your total cholesterol is 220 and your HDL number turns out to be 22, your ratio of total to HDL cholesterol is roughly 10 to 1. A total/HDL ratio greater than 5 to 1 is usually connected with increased risk. However, if your HDL were 88, that same ratio would be only 2.5, definitely putting you in the favorable, or low-risk, category. Obviously, without the HDL figure, the total of 220 remains ambiguous and yields incomplete information.

A new, potentially more accurate "apolipoprotein" test has recently been added to our arsenal of heart-disease predictors. So far, research using the test is preliminary but promising; early results show that it may have greater prognostic value than the traditional cholesterol/HDL measurements. Right now, the test is available from many nutrition-minded physicians, and it is not costly to perform.

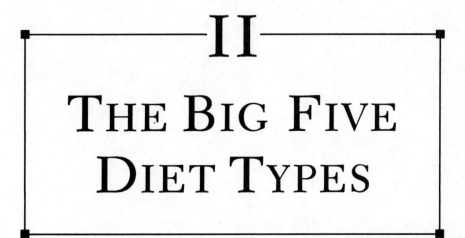

II

THE BIG FIVE
DIET TYPES

In this part of the book, start by reading the special section that pertains to you, based on your answers to the questionnaire. For example, if the majority of your responses indicate that you're a Diet Type 2—a good candidate for the Modified Protein-Plus Diet—head directly for that part first. However, crucial information and guidelines that apply to *all* the Diet Types are found in the sections on Diet Types 1, 4 and 5, which spell out the newest findings and offer practical advice on fiber and complex carbohydrates, fresh fruit and vegetables and "convenience" foods, respectively. Since the Protein-Plus plan involves all these elements, the three additional sections are a "must read" to complete the picture.

The exception is Diet Type 3. The only people who need to consult this chapter are those with already diagnosed or suspected food-based allergies, which the questionnaire should help you identify. (If you are a Type 3, you should turn to all the other sections, too, of course.)

Another good reason for reading the material outside your own Diet Type is that the questionnaire is weighted (as has already been explained.) That means you may have come up with a number of answers that place you partly in other categories. While you probably have a clear-cut or even overwhelming majority of responses in one section, some of you may also turn out to be a mix of types. From my practice, I've found that if there are any overlaps, they will most likely occur between Diet Types 1 and 4 —both stress a high-carbohydrate approach, though each has a different emphasis —and Types 2 and 5, both of which tend to attract a more mainstream, "balanced" dieter.

Chapter 9, "How to Stay Slim on Any Diet," will focus on behavioral strategies that are relevant to all the Diet Types. These tactics should help reinforce the initial results you achieve and lay the groundwork for lasting weight control and well-being.

Each of the five Diet Type menus and their accompanying set of recipes should serve as a general guideline. Follow a given diet as is, or use it to design your own eating plan as well as to help you select restaurant or take-out meals. Also, be flexible. Consider substituting corresponding dishes from any of the other Diet Types. For quick, easy alternatives, consult the "Five Easy Pieces" provided for each diet. Keep in mind that these slimming, well-varied food plans should serve as a model for healthful eating habits that last beyond the featured seven days.

The nutritionally balanced, well-varied sample menu plan you will select is designed to help you lose weight and then to maintain your desired weight once you reach it. It features a rich selection of delicious and sustaining low-fat foods and recipes that we hope will serve as inspiration for future weeks. Feel free to substitute other foods from the same category using the suggestions offered in the chapter pertaining to both your own Diet Type and the other Diet Type chapters and menus. Once you approach the ideal weight for your body, your inner diet "thermostat" will automatically make adjustments to help you level off. If you find you are not losing weight or become "stuck" for any length of time, increase your level of aerobic activity before you consider cutting your food portions. Refer back to Chapter 2 for the indispensable benefits of exercise and why undereating can make you fatter. Above all, don't start this diet before thoroughly reading the material covered in the chapter that refers to your chosen Diet Type as well as all the others.

Each of the diets is roughly 1,200 calories. But more important than their quantity is their *quality:* They are low in fats, sugar, sodium and cholesterol; low to moderate in animal protein; and rich in fiber and important carbohydrates— a formula essential to lasting slimness and health. Remember, these diets are not intended to be one-week or one-month regimens, but rather lifetime plans that you can modify and vary with the help of the ample information offered throughout the book. Note the patterns of each diet, the portion sizes given for grains, vegetables, fruits, dairy foods and meats, so you can create a similar program with other foods within each of these groups that are equally nutritious and low in fat. *To gain more weight or slow down weight loss, increase portion sizes of all foods except fats and animal proteins.*

To help you design your own menus, note the following rough equivalents:

CARBOHYDRATES

4 ounces or ½ cup brown rice or any cooked whole grain = ½ cup whole-wheat pasta = 1 slice whole-grain bread = 1 medium or ¾ cup starchy vegetable (such as potatoes, squash, corn) = ½ cup legumes.

1 cup raw vegetables = ½ cup cooked

1 medium fruit = ½ cup pureed fresh fruit = ¾ cup berries = ½ cup fresh-squeezed juice

PROTEIN/ DAIRY

2 ounces 1 percent fat or dry-curd cottage cheese = 1 cup skim milk = ¾ cup plain low- or nonfat yogurt = 1 ounce hard, part-skim cheese

ANIMAL/SOY

4 ounces fish, lean poultry or meat = 6 ounces tofu or any soy protein food

4

DIET TYPE 1

The High-Fiber/ Super Grain Diet

George Burns once offered this opinion of the high-fiber diet plan: "Fiber? You can't knock it. Have you ever seen a fat moth?"

Ironically, one of the most beneficial components of your diet is hardly even digestible. It's also had the best press ever enjoyed by any food. The much praised fiber, once known less reverently as "roughage," is now considered protective against both heart disease and certain forms of cancer, as well as a proven remedy for a number of intestinal complaints.

While fiber fervor may seem of recent origin, this unassuming edible has actually been held in high esteem since the time of Hippocrates (around 400 B.C.), who recommended plenty of wheat-grain bread, vegetables and fruits for healthy bowels. In the 1830s, fiery American evangelist Sylvester Graham—for whom the graham cracker was named—touted the virtues of bran and vegetarianism from his Sunday pulpit. Later in the century, Seventh-Day Adventist physician Dr. John Harvey Kellogg, who ran a well-heeled sanatorium in Battle Creek, Michigan, held that all disease stemmed from toxins in the intestines and advocated a special purifying regimen, or "nature's broom" diet, of cabbage, carrots, corn, potatoes, steel-cut oats and bran, among other wholesome staples, to sweep them away. By the 1890s his patented breakfast cereals were already becoming a national institution.

In the early 1900s, however, fiber fell into general disfavor, as a new generation of doctors blamed it for bowel irritation, cramps, ulcers, indigestion and bloating, and even for serious inflammatory conditions such as diverticulosis. At the same time, the pristine-looking white bread, stripped of its coarse dark bran and other whole-grain trappings, was becoming the trendy alternative for millions of Americans who somehow came to equate refined white flour with progress and civilization.

Then in the 1970s, fiber was rediscovered. A British research group led by Dr. Denis Burkitt, a noted surgeon, observed that the incidence of colon cancer, heart disease, diabetes and obesity, among other typical Western ills, was rare in certain developing countries of Africa. Why? The African groups ate extremely fibrous diets rich in grains, nuts, seeds and wild plants, and low in milk and meat fats, while Americans and northern Europeans tended toward an excess of processed, low-fiber, high-fat foods. Dr. Burkitt held that the standard Western diet slows movement of food though the intestines, keeping potential cancer-promoting chemicals in the digestive tract too long. Other studies eventually confirmed his findings, restoring fiber to its former status.

Today, high-fiber diets, incarnated in such recent bestsellers as *The F-Plan Diet* and *The Pritikin Program for Diet and Exercise*, are considered both a safeguard against major disease and a healthy, dramatically effective way to lose weight. They have also been credited with helping to reverse as well as prevent certain disorders.

As a result, the demand for fiber has reached record levels, and virtually every box of breakfast cereal now tries to lure buyers with the promise of plenty. The popularity of carbohydrates, fiber's digestible companion, is also at an all-time high. If we haven't yet overhauled our national eating habits, at least we're paying more "lip service" to these wholesome foods.

WHAT'S A CARBOHYDRATE?

Energy is the body's number-one demand and carbohydrates are its favorite fuel—the most efficient raw material available to all cells, including those of your muscles, brain and nervous system. Unlike proteins or fats, carbohydrates burn "clean," which means they are converted to energy (glucose) without leaving behind any toxic residues; the only wastes they produce are carbon dioxide and water, both easily released though natural processes like breathing and perspiration. The body has to work a lot harder to break down the more complex fats and proteins to service its cells, and has a much bigger cleanup job afterward, too.

Carbohydrates come in two varieties: the sugars, or "simple" carbohydrates and the starches, or "complex" kind. In their natural, unrefined, unprocessed state, the vast majority of complex and simple carbohydrates come well-endowed with essential nutrients and hunger-appeasing fiber, and are low in fat and calories, too. Consider the wholesome roundup: fresh, unpeeled fruits; whole-grain breads, cereals and flours, such as wheat, corn, rice, rye and oats; pastas; potatoes; beans and peas (legumes); fresh vegetables; and dairy foods. The last are the only carbohydrates lacking in fiber. Dairy foods and many other carbohydrates are also rich sources of protein (see Diet Type 2). It's the refined, adulterated carbohydrates—cakes, pastries, candies, cookies, ice cream, all laced with fat and sugar and robbed of nutrients— that have given the bona fide ones a bad reputation. They're also notoriously short on fiber, so it's easy to overeat them.

FIBER FIGHTS FAT

In 1910, Americans on the average were a lot leaner than they are now—and they consumed a good deal more bread and cereal, fresh vegetables and fruits, along with far less meat and sugar. But until very recently, few of us would have made the connection between high-fiber foods and slimness. In fact, you could always spot dieters by the absence of bread, pasta or potatoes on their plate, and by their panic at the mention of "starch." By removing the bun from the burger or swearing off the potato that comes with the steak, they thought they were prudently cutting back on fattening calories.

But plenty of carbohydrates in your diet can actually *enhance* your efforts to lose weight. This radical-sounding notion was put to a convincing test in a recent study at Michigan State University. After eight weeks, a group of overweight men eating twelve slices of a high-fiber bread every day along with their three regular, moderate-calorie meals lost an average of nearly 20 pounds! Those eating a low-fiber bread lost 13.7 pounds. How is this possible?

For one thing, carbohydrates have the same number of calories per ounce as protein, and fewer than half as many as fat. What's more, they're naturally filling and keep a lively appetite in check. The Michigan researchers concluded that because the subjects ate bread with each meal, they became satisfied before they consumed their usual quota of calories. A study by the U.S. Department of Agriculture showed that simply adding a moderate amount of fiber to a meal actually decreases the number of calories the body absorbs from it. And in other experiments, animals who were fed an equal number of calories (and did the same amount of exercise) lost weight at different rates. Apparently, their food source was the deciding factor: Those who were given fat weighed the most, and those fed protein were the next highest on the scale. Animals eating carbohydrates, however, ended up the thinnest! Even if you *overindulge* in complex carbohydrates, the body may compensate by raising the metabolic rate—a response that is apparently not triggered when you eat large amounts of protein or fat.

Besides conserving calories, most complex carbohydrates carry a rich load of vitamins, minerals, trace elements and low-fat vegetable proteins. The forbidden baked potato on the dieter's plate contains only about one-fifth the calories of the medium-sized steak, none of the fat and cholesterol, and offers a wealth of nutrients into the bargain, including iron, protein, thiamine, niacin, vitamin C, phosphorus, iodine, vitamin B-6, copper, magnesium and folic acid. The only fattening things about a potato are the butter and sour cream traditionally used to flavor it; try plain yogurt or low-fat cottage cheese with freshly ground pepper, chopped dill and parsley or scallions, and you have a diet food par excellence.

Potatoes in their skins, grainy foods like bread and cereal, and crunchy fresh fruits and vegetables are psychologically satisfying because they require a lot of chewing and take a good while to eat. They also release their calories at a steady, manageable rate. In another study, ten healthy people at Great Britain's Bristol University were given either an apple, applesauce or apple juice—all equivalent in calorie content. Since the apple took the longest time to eat, it was reported to be the most filling, followed by the sauce and juice. While everyone's blood sugar rose an equal amount, the increase in the output of insulin, the hormone that converts sugar into fat, was twice as high after the juice as it was after the apple. A few hours after the apple meal, the blood sugar level registered normal, whereas it fell to *below* normal following the juice and the sauce.

The implication for dieters is dramatic: The high-fiber apple held off hunger the longest and it kept the blood sugar relatively stable. However, the fiber-deficient juice left people feeling the hungriest; by forcing the release of so much insulin, it led to a temporary sugar shortage, or what is called "reactive hypoglycemia" (see p. 86). As this simple experiment suggests, a fiber-rich diet is ideal for overweight people as well as diabetics, since it apparently regulates blood sugar and appetite and reduces the body's requirement for insulin.

LONGEVITY FOODS

During World War I Denmark was forced to transform its traditional eating habits—and the consequences are hard to dismiss as mere happenstance. A blockade by the Germans cut off much of the nation's food supply, including the grain that fed its pigs, cattle and chickens. To conserve more of the precious wheat for its citizens, the country's food advisor ordered much of its livestock killed. The intake of pork and other meats as well as milk and butter dramatically declined, and the Danish population relied more on whole-grain cereals, fresh vegetables, legumes and fruits—becoming the healthiest country in Europe. Denmark's death rate due to heart disease dropped by 60 percent and the overall death rate by 40 percent. Unfortunately, the statistics rose quickly to their preblockade levels when the people resumed their normal (high-fat, low-fiber) diet after the war.

Coincidence? Hardly. Diets high in complex carbohydrates are the only ones not associated with any killer diseases. By contrast, diets high in fat and animal protein and low in fiber have been linked with our most common disorders, particularly heart and blood-vessel disease. Even polyunsaturates may have a damaging effect on artery walls because they encourage the clumping of red blood cells along with formation of free radicals, "terrorist" molecules that are randomly destructive to delicate cell membranes.

But fats are not the only source of trouble. Highly refined sugars and starches also raise blood lipids (fats) by releasing calories in the form of glucose too rapidly into the bloodstream. When we eat any carbohydrate, the body summons tiny glands in the pancreas to secrete insulin, which allows glucose to pass into the cell either for use as energy or storage as fat. But when the food consists mostly of processed sugar and flour and lacks fiber—cake or pastry, for example —it's as if the body were given a large injection of glucose all at once, and insulin has to be stepped up sharply to meet the sudden demand. Excess insulin "eats up" too much sugar, causing glucose levels to drop very low for a while before returning to normal. This response, known as reactive hypoglycemia, is exactly what happened in the apple/apple juice study, and it explains why people often feel hungry, irritable and drained of energy soon after eating sweets.

During the interval when the insulin overracts and blood sugar is in scant supply, the body favors the buildup of *triglycerides*—circulating fats in the blood that are one of the key factors in heart disease. Just as with cholesterol, people (especially women) with a high triglyceride level are at greater risk for heart attacks and strokes.

Unlike their refined cousins, however, high-fiber complex carbohydrates are turned into glucose at a slower, steadier rate. This means no surplus of insulin is released to use up the blood's available sugar and encourage high levels of fats. This keeps the dangerous blood lipids and fatty acids under control, thus protecting the heart and maintaining an even supply of energy.

FIBER COUNTS!

A recent study in Bristol, England, showed that the blood glucose levels in ten healthy volunteers rose higher and then fell more sharply after a meal of processed snack foods such as a candy bar, a cola drink and potato chips, than after consumption of whole foods such as raisins, peanuts and bananas. Evidently, blood-sugar levels are more unstable and carbohydrates are consumed more rapidly following a sweetened, fiber-deficient snack. One woman showed a pathological drop in blood sugar (hypoglycemia) after eating the processed foods but had a normal blood-sugar response after eating the whole-food snack.

DON'T OVERDO IT!

I used to think that fat in the blood invariably stemmed from dietary fat. A woman patient of mine once beautifully illustrated that this was not always the case. Because she had high circulating blood fats (triglycerides), I placed her on a high-fiber diet, virtually eliminating fat. She came back two months later with practically the same high triglyceride level, and I accused her of cheating with her fat consumption. She vehemently denied using any fats, but admitted to substituting large quantities of fresh fruit and several quarts of natural fruit juice for her high-fat treats. Once she eliminated fruits and juices, her triglycerides plummeted to normal levels. The fact is that *excess calories from any sugar*, even the natural kind found in fresh fruit, may be converted easily into artery-clogging triglycerides.

In one study, ten patients with high triglyceride levels reduced these amounts by 63 percent during the first ten days on a high-fiber diet and by 91 percent after six months. They achieved these results without losing any weight simply by consuming up to 50 grams of dietary fiber from oat bran every day.

Fiber-rich carbohydrates also absorb cholesterol, hastening its elimination by the body. They soak up bile acids and intestinal carcinogens, too, which shields the colon from cancer. And they encourage the growth of certain colon organisms that crowd out dangerous, tumor-promoting bacteria.

You won't find complete protection packed into one miracle food: A combination of different forms of fiber is the body's best medicine. All fibers fall into one of two categories. The soft, mucousy, spongelike (soluble) kind absorbs

water (and often fats), swelling in size, slowing down digestion and making you feel fuller longer. The harder, grittier
(insoluble) kind also slows digestion in the stomach, but acts
more like a fast-moving pipe cleaner in the intestines, speeding up the time it takes for food to pass through them and
whisking away potential cancer-causing agents before they
have a chance to do any mischief. Both types of fiber promote
the growth of beneficial bacteria within the body.

Apples, grapes, prunes, citrus fruits, corn, potatoes and
squash all contain pectin, a "soft," soluble fiber that holds
water and fats and prevents radical shifts in blood sugar. Peas
and beans, oatmeal, oat bran and barley have the same effect.
Eaten regularly, such foods also lower blood cholesterol and
help control diabetes. One recent experiment showed that
adding just one bowl of oat bran cereal and five oat bran
muffins a day to an otherwise standard American diet reduced cholesterol an average of 13 percent after just ten days,
and almost 20 percent within three weeks. One and a half
cups of cooked navy and pinto beans daily had the same
effect.

If you've ever added wheat bran to your morning cereal,
then you've probably noticed that it doesn't dissolve. Behav-
ing the same way inside your digestive tract, this coarse,
chewy substance helps step up the passage of food through
your system so the body has little chance of exposure to possibly harmful chemicals and impurities. Whole-grain breads
and cereals, along with such cruciferous and root vegetables
as turnips, broccoli, brussels sprouts, cabbage, beets and carrots, also quicken your food's transit time, as well as absorbing fats and cholesterol. Most populations with high-fiber
diets and low rates of cancer, such as the rural Finns and
Danes, eat a lot of breads and cereals containing insoluble
fiber.

Not surprisingly, vegetarians with high-fiber diets have
lower fat, cholesterol and blood-pressure levels and lower
rates of colon and rectal cancer than those who consume less
than 10 grams of fiber a day. They also have less frequent
bowel problems, diverticular disease and hemorrhoids.

It appears fiber may help prevent breast cancer, too: A study of over 1,400 healthy women in San Francisco found that those who were chronically constipated (and presumably on low-fiber diets) were more likely to have abnormal cells in their breast fluid than those with regular bowel functions.

Estrogen levels are also lower in women who eat plenty of fiber and complex carbohydrates than in those whose diets are high in animal protein and low in fiber. Fibrous foods apparently bind the hormone and facilitate its passage out of the body. That's good news, since excess estrogen can increase the risk of breast and endometrial cancer, uterine fibroids, endometriosis and premenstrual syndrome.

We have already seen how high-fiber diets can make the body less dependent on insulin. As reported recently in the *Journal of Clinical Nutrition,* Australian aborigines, like the Pima Indians in the United States, are prone to diabetes, especially when they move to an urban setting and adopt "Western"-type diets. However, their blood sugar can often be brought back to normal once they resume their former eating habits. Their native cuisine is so fibrous, it makes brown rice look like Häagen-Dazs ice cream by comparison! The aborigines eat such foods as "bramble-wattles," reeds and plant shoots, which sometimes require days of slow cooking, soaking, boiling or pounding to make them edible at all. The high fiber content of these foods acts as a time-release mechanism to deliver sugars very slowly into the digestive tract—ideal nourishment for diabetics. Guar gum, a form of soluble fiber from which pasta can be made, has also been shown to stabilize blood sugar very effectively in diabetics because of its similar "slow-release" properties.

HOW MUCH DO YOU NEED?

If a food claims to be high in a certain nutrient, such as vitamin C, FDA regulations require that it contain at least 10 percent of the U.S. Recommended Dietary Allowance (RDA) for that nutrient. However, no comparable ground rules have yet been set for fiber. That means there is no minimum a cereal must have to make any label claims. What's a reasonable amount? A food should contain at least 2.5 to 3 grams of fiber to deserve billing as a "good" source.

On the average, Americans now consume about 15 grams of fiber a day. To derive any benefits comparable to those enjoyed in non-Western countries, you should double (and preferably triple) that number. This calls for eating reasonable portions throughout the day—never all at one meal—to ensure that you're eating different types of fiber with all their special advantages.

Until recently, scientists resorted to an awkward and misleading method to determine the amount of fiber in foods. They gave the food in question a real going-over, first by soaking it in a strong chemical solvent, then treating it with hot acids and alkalis; whatever remained intact after this assault was presumed to be the indigestible component, or "crude" fiber. But much dietary fiber was destroyed in the process. In fact, foods may contain up to seven times more fiber than the "crude" figure would suggest. Fortunately, methods of content analysis have since been greatly improved.

You may have heard the warnings that too much fiber can interfere with the absorption of certain nutrients, especially zinc, iron, calcium and magnesium. While this is partly true, it happens only if you eat excessive amounts of bran-enriched wheat bread or cereal at every meal or add refined fiber to an otherwise nutrition-poor diet. Besides, fiber foods are often rich in minerals, especially zinc, which can help compensate for any nutrient loss. Also, as you eat more complex carbohydrates and fewer animal proteins, your need for calcium and other minerals actually decreases. This is because an oversupply of protein causes minerals such as calcium and zinc to be excreted in your urine, while no such loss occurs on diets that are either moderate or low in protein.

For fiber's sake, don't add too much to your diet too *soon*. Bloating, flatulence, cramps and diarrhea are common com-

FIBER FACT: WHY YOU CAN'T DIGEST IT

Foods rich in complex carbohydrates and fiber, such as grains and beans, often contain digestion-inhibiting enzymes because they originally come from seeds. In the wild, animals relocate to new territories by crawling, walking, flying or swimming. Since plants aren't mobile, however, their seeds have to "hitch a ride" from one place to another. Some, such as the dandelion, have evolved fluffy "feathers" that allow them to be wind-borne; some have burrs that stick to the fur of animals and are carried hundreds of miles on their backs. But others have evolved a different strategy. They look and taste enticing enough to be eaten by herbivorous animals. Nature has cleverly made these seeds indigestible so that they're transported a certain distance inside the animals' digestive tracts, then eliminated intact and dropped onto the ground, where they find a new place to grow.

Thus, fiber foods' natural indigestibility is a means of transportation and survival. While beans, seeds and grains—mainstays of any high-carbohydrate, high-fiber diet—will all to some degree resist digestion, you *can* fight back. For example, thoroughly soaking or sprouting beans and seeds (see p. 248) will enhance their digestibility, as will cooking them with a seaweed called kombu (available at health-food stores and Oriental groceries), which blocks their digestion inhibitors. Another strategy for "degassing" beans: pour off and replace the boiling water several times during the cooking process.

Chewing high-fiber foods well is also crucial, since all digestion begins in the mouth: Don't gobble crunchy bran cereal or brown rice the same way you would a jelly doughnut!

plaints of those who make the sudden switch from, say, sugar doughnuts and black coffee to six heaping tablespoons of bran on whole wheat cereal for breakfast. Fiber is basically left alone by your digestive juices until it reaches the colon, or large intestine. There it is set upon by intestinal bacteria and the resulting fermentation releases various kinds of gas. It takes several weeks for your bacteria to adjust to the presence of added fiber and for the gas to subside. So take it easy at first and increase your intake gradually, or else the discomfort may drive you back to your former eating habits. And remember, don't just pour on the bran. The benefits of a variety of fibers complement each other, and you'll need them all for optimum health.

Most important, never use fiber to give you a false sense of security about the rest of your diet. Adding wheat or oat bran to your thickly buttered, syrup-sweetened, refined-flour pancakes will not automatically make them wholesome or justify otherwise careless eating. (For a list of some high-fiber foods, see pages 316-317.)

Since most of the foods on the high-fiber, high-carbohydrate diet are low in calories and abundant in water and bulk, you don't have to worry about measuring portions to the ounce (healthy overindulgence is permitted!). In fact, most of the vegetables can be eaten in "unlimited" amounts. The foods have built-in satiety value, which means you should automatically stop eating at about the right point.

If you're a nibbler or the type who always keeps something around to munch on, you generally like to decide when and how to eat and may have a hard time with an overly structured eating plan. If you tend to eat more than usual when you're lonely, anxious or bored, or must chew on something frequently, your best choices are fiber-rich foods that have a high nutrient-to-calorie ratio. Diet Type 1 permits enough snacking throughout the day to appease even the most tenacious appetites and to help prevent overeating at scheduled meals.

Since complex carbohydrates are your body's most readily usable source of energy, Diet Type 1 is tailor-made for the physically active. If you jog or take aerobic dance at least three times a week or are a sports enthusiast, you will benefit from the steady-burning fuel that only high-fiber nutrition can provide.

Be aware that any diet rich in grains and beans will definitely call for more shopping, preparation and cooking time than usual. This may be unwelcome news for work-weary types with hectic routines who can't handle anything more strenuous than opening a can after arriving home. Unfortunately, canning and freezing often lower vitamin and mineral content. However, some beans such as lentils and split peas don't require soaking and cook rather quickly, and grains such as bulgur, cream of rice and barley are precooked or simple to prepare. For other beans, a pressure cooker can

THE SUPER ENERGY DIET

The much-admired Tarahumara Indians of northwestern Mexico's Sierra Madre mountains live almost entirely on a diet of beans, corn, squash, pumpkins, root vegetables, wild plants, fruit and about 1 percent animal food. They show incredible endurance and strength; almost none are obese. With their sturdy, wiry bodies, the Tarahumaras make superb, Olympic-caliber runners. In their tribal pastime, a soccerlike sport played with an oak ball the size of a baseball, they run a total of two hundred miles before finishing the game. During the night, other player/runners light the course's way with torches, stopping for a break only every twelve miles or so!

Think about it: Studies have found that people on a high-fat diet could do strenuous exercise for only an hour. But on a high-carbohydrate diet, they could perform the very same workload for up to *four* hours.

shorten preparation time considerably, and vegetables can easily be stir-fried or steamed. Quick-fix guidelines and recipes are included for those who are especially short on time or patience.

This diet may pose problems for people with allergies to grains or for those with inordinate cravings for starchy, high-calorie carbohydrates. Overweight women are more likely than men to be carbohydrate sensitive, or prone to retaining fluids when they eat too many of these foods. Even on a healthy, high-carbohydrate diet, the pounds such people lose in the form of fat may be canceled out by added water weight —and the frustrating holding pattern may last for a week or even a few months. Others have an unusual craving for carbohydrates and gain weight simply because they overeat them.

Studies by Dr. Judith Wurtman at Michigan State University reveal that there may be a definite biochemical basis for such a craving. Such people reportedly have low levels of serotonin, the brain chemical that monitors moods and sleep, among other body functions. Consequences of this deficiency include sleeplessness, irritability, moodiness and depression. One of serotonin's building blocks is L-tryptophan, an amino acid found in certain protein foods. Eating such foods alone, however, does not allow the tryptophan to cross the blood/brain barrier where it can be absorbed and converted to serotonin, because the other amino acids in proteins compete with it. Carbohydrates, however, promote tryptophan's absorption and conversion, and thus bring about a sense of calm, well-being and even euphoria.

Many women with premenstrual syndrome have lower-than-normal serotonin levels and are carbohydrate cravers. Predictably, their cravings are often preceded by periods of tension and restlessness, and the tryptophan-boosting carbohydrates have a relaxing, antidepressant effect.

Under a doctor's guidance, many carbohydrate cravers can be treated with moderate amounts of tryptophan supplements (available in health-food stores). These can reduce their overdependence on carbohydrate foods for the mood-elevating chemical and help them break their addictive pattern.

Some doctors believe that because of their special needs, overweight carbohydrate cravers should have generous amounts of carbohydrates in their diets. But this may be like allowing former alcoholics to indulge in liquor at parties, and it could set the stage for trouble. In my practice I have found that such people often fare very well on protein-dominant diets (see Diet Type 2), since they are not as often exposed to the kinds of foods that make them feel so good and tempt them to overeat in the first place.

Regardless of which diet plan works best for you, the most important point is to be aware that carbohydrate cravings *do* exist and can be a powerful influence on your eating behavior, including the foods you choose for a snack or binge. They may also explain why you have had difficulty with certain diets in the past. As with so much else, knowing about this condition is the first step in learning how to overcome it.

Exotic or ethnic ingredients that give high-fiber, high-carbohydrate diets taste appeal and even the basic ingredients of macrobiotic cuisine may be hard to find in some places. It's also a challenge to stick to this kind of eating plan while you're traveling or on the run. Some variations on this Diet Type have been needlessly restrictive. As you might recall, the commendable high-fiber Pritikin program was extremely low in fat; in fact many people found it too drastic to be palatable for long.

The latest research reveals that such a rigid moratorium on fats is not only unnecessary but may actually be a disadvantage. Along with helping you feel satisfied, healthy fats, such as the Omega-3 fatty acids found in seafood, as well as the monounsaturated oils like olive and soy, may be protective in themselves. The Mediterranean peoples, the Eskimos and the Japanese, whose diets are high in one or both types of fat, show a markedly lower rate of coronary heart disease and certain cancers, particularly of the breast and colon. The good oils apparently inhibit the production of certain harmful prostaglandins, natural hormonelike substances which

CARBOHYDRATE CRAVING:
SWEET TOOTH OR ... FAT TOOTH?

In a recent experiment, overweight individuals were divided into two groups according to their snacking behavior. Those who reached for such goodies as Snickers® bars, date-nut granola cookies and peanut-cream patties were labeled carbohydrate cravers. In contrast, those who didn't indulge in these items were the protein types, preferring such choices as lean corned beef wrapped around cream cheese, beef jerky and boiled ham between meals.

Carbohydrate cravers were by far the more numerous group. Out of seventy overweight subjects, fifty-one, or 73 percent, ate mostly carbohydrate-rich snack foods. However, nutritional analysis of these foods has shown that most are mixtures of sugar and fat. While a "sweet tooth" is a preference for sugary treats, candy and other desserts, many such foods are often higher in fat than in carbohydrates—and it is calories from the former that may more readily lead to unwanted body fat. (See also Chapter 2, pages 24-25.)

may play a role in tumor formation and blood coagulation. In addition, these beneficial fats reduce the amount of harmful cholesterol, the kind that deposits fat on artery walls, in the blood while preserving or increasing the healthy kind, high-density lipoproteins, or HDLs, which isolate and remove harmful cholesterol from the body.

In a recent study at the Agricultural University in the Netherlands, a high-carbohydrate diet with a generous intake of total fat in the form of olive oil but little saturated fat turned out to be more heart-protective than the very-low-fat, high-carbohydrate diet traditionally recommended for heart

COMPATIBLE CARBOHYDRATES

Scientists believe that the human body evolved into its present state at a time when man was primarily a hunter-gatherer subsisting on nuts, grains, seeds and fruits, and when large protein-containing meals were sporadic at best (whenever he successfully hunted wild game). Thus, our digestive tracts and metabolism were designed to be compatible with high-fiber, high-carbohydrate foods, while retaining the flexibility to handle occasional high-protein meals.

patients. Beneficial HDL levels rose slightly on the olive-oil-rich diet but fell on the low-fat plan; harmful triglycerides, however, dropped by a significant amount on the "fatty" diet and increased on the ultra-lean one.

One of my patients, meticulous and responsible about his weight and health, took up a Pritikin-type regimen on his own to correct his high-cholesterol condition. He started out with 245 milligrams in his bloodstream and, sure enough, after six weeks on this high-fiber, almost zero-added-fat diet, his cholesterol dropped to 200. Bravo! However, at the same time, his triglycerides rose from 100 to 160. What had gone wrong? Apparently, an excess of carbohydrates, including nutritious fruits, can raise triglycerides. What my not-quite-healthy patient's diet lacked was fish and olive oils, either of which can keep triglycerides under control. After adding them (and reducing fruits), his cholesterol dropped to 165, and his triglycerides restablized at 100. Thus, adding small amounts of one or both these oils can turn an almost-wholesome diet into a superlative and probably safer one.

Incidentally, researchers have recently discovered that a high level of triglycerides *by itself* forecasts heart disease in women, even when their cholesterol levels are normal. (In

WHATEVER HAPPENED TO HYPOGLYCEMIA?

Hypoglycemia, or low blood sugar, was a much-publicized condition in the late 1960s and '70s, but the medical profession largely dismissed it as a trendy diagnosis referring to a relative handful of patients. However, the concept recently resurfaced with high credibility, thanks to a group of researchers at Johns Hopkins University School of Medicine and the National Institutes of Health who renamed the condition "idiopathic postprandial syndrome," or IPS. Normally, people with this disorder would complain to their doctors of such symptoms as irritability, tension, fatigue, palpitations and cold hands, conditions that would be relieved temporarily by eating sweets. However, when their doctors checked their blood sugar via a glucose tolerance test they found no abnormally low readings, and so attributed the symptoms to some other problem—or to just plain neurosis!

Fortunately, the Johns Hopkins scientists measured not only blood sugar but also levels of adrenaline, cortisol and growth hormone, all chemicals which defend the body's sugar level and try to keep it in balance. In patients complaining of IPS, they found that amounts of all three substances, especially the "fight or flight" hormone adrenaline, were abnormally high. Sure enough, the output of such chemicals increases whenever the blood sugar drops too low, since they act to compensate for any shortage. This is the reason doctors could find no real drop in blood sugar via traditional tests: The three compounds were quickly sounding an alarm and rushing in to maintain a state of equilibrium. Adrenaline is responsible for the symptoms of nervous irritability, sweaty palms, palpitations and even panic that typically accompany the syndrome.

(Continued)

(Continued)

This experiment establishes that IPS is a recogniz-
able medical problem and that the blood sugar count
alone is an inadequate or outright misleading index.
Now doctors have a more thorough and sophisticated
way to ensure the right diagnosis.

If you turn out to be hypoglycemic, your doctor has
the choice of recommending either a diet high in complex carbohydrates (preferably spread over several
small meals a day, rather than three "square" ones) or
a protein-rich plan, since both are effective in stabiliz-
ing blood sugar.

---

men, both cholesterol and triglyceride readings must be elevated to indicate a true heart-disease risk.)

With some creative revising and rethinking, it's possible
to resolve the drawbacks of the Pritikin and other high-
carbohydrate-type diets with which you may already be
familiar. The result is Diet Type 1, aimed at those whose
responses to the questionnaire have placed them in this category. Check out the following roundup of the "Super Carbohydrates" for a more detailed look at some of the staples
on Diet Type 1, then turn to the sample seven-day eating
plan. Follow it exactly as is, or use it as a guideline to help
you design the most appealing and convenient diet for you
and your family.

THE SUPER CARBOHYDRATES

WHEAT: Almost every diet throughout the world is based on
a grain. For example, rice rules in China and Japan, bulgur
holds sway in the Middle East, while pasta dominates in
Italy, rye and buckwheat in Russia and corn in Mexico. Millet, barley and oats are other ethnic staples. Unfortunately,
the steel rolling mill, invented just over a hundred years ago,
ushered in the era of modern processing, stripping grains of
most of their vitamins, minerals, fiber and trace elements, all
in the name of progress. Wheat flour was bleached, rice pol-

ished, corn degerminated and barley pearled. Processing wheat to make white flour removes most of the chromium, manganese, iron, copper, zinc, magnesium and a host of vitamins—thiamine, riboflavin, niacin, pyridoxine, pantothenic acid, folic acid (all members of the B complex) and vitamin E and essential fatty acids. Enrichment restores only part of this nutritional treasure and none of the fiber.

About 80 percent of wheat's essential nutrients and almost all its fiber are stored in the bran and germ, both of which are entirely removed from the kernel when flour is milled or refined. However, when the wheat grain is stone-ground, the bran and germ are left intact. Health-food stores sell bread made from a variety of grains, most of them stone-ground, and baked without the dubious hydrogenated vegetable oils or shortenings or high-sodium preservatives typical of most regular supermarket breads. One of the more wholesome varieties consists entirely of sprouted grains like wheat, barley, millet, rye, corn and whole oats, along with lentils, soybeans and a sprinkling of sea salt—delicious!

Right now, the best supermarket choices include whole-grain pita or "pocket" bread, fiber-added Roman Meal, Sunbeam, Weight Watchers, Wonder or Thomas's "Lite" wheat, cracked wheat and white breads and whole-grain bagels, all without shortening and lower in calories than standard store-bought breads. Those with allergies to wheat and/or other grains should consult Diet Type 3 for a fuller list.

The same rule applies to cereals: The least processed kinds are best. These include whole-grain hot varieties, such as Wheatena, whole (noninstant) or steel-cut oats, oat bran and rye, buckwheat and brown-rice cereal. Among the cold cereals, Kellogg's All-Bran with Extra Fiber, General Mills Fiber One and Nabisco Shredded Wheat 'n Bran are the richest in fiber, as their names suggest, although only the third has no added sugar or other sweeteners. Cheerios and Gerber's Toasted Oat Cereal, made entirely from oats, are good sources of protein, and both are low in calories and sodium. Try adding a tablespoon or two each of wheat and oat bran to these or any cold or hot grain cereals for more fiber.

Beware of packaged granolas: While their base of rolled oats, seeds and nuts presents a wholesome image, they're drizzled with refined sugar in the form of honey or molasses, along with coconut oil, which is more saturated than beef fat! One serving packs a whopping 500 calories. Better to use granola as a topping for a dash of flavor, or to make your own (see recipe, p. 109).

RICE: This is basic to the dishes of many countries—Indian curries, Spanish paellas, Italian risottos, Greek kabobs. Just as with bread, white, refined, polished rice is a pale nutritional shadow—stripped of B vitamins, fiber and protein—of the whole, brown original. The nutty-flavored brown rice breaks down into glucose at a gradual rate of about 2 calories a minute. (By contrast, a candy bar yields 30 calories a minute.) This slow release keeps insulin from being overproduced and sending the body into a temporary sugar/energy shortage. Brown rice releases sugar more slowly than potatoes and other carbohydrate foods, which is why it appears often on diets recommended for diabetics. Short-, medium- and long-grain are equally nutritious, providing potassium, selenium and magnesium, among other important minerals.

Note: If you prefer white rice, buy the enriched parboiled or converted kind for maximum nutrition and avoid instant or "minute" varieties.

BULGUR: Also known as cracked wheat, and a good source of potassium and fiber, this is a favorite in Middle Eastern cooking. For example, tabouli is a piquant blend of cracked wheat, olive oil, chopped tomatoes, onion and parsley, a tasty side dish or appetizer often served with whole-wheat pita bread. You can find bulgur in Middle Eastern or gourmet specialty shops, supermarkets and health-food stores.

BUCKWHEAT (KASHA): Strictly speaking, buckwheat is not a grain, since it's from the flower of a cereal plant, not its seed. But throughout history it has been eaten as a cereal, used the same way as rye, oats, rice, wheat and millet. The kernels are ground into a coarse meal known as kasha, and the result is a food rich in protein, iron, potassium and B complex vitamins. In supermarkets, kasha can usually be found in the rice or gourmet section.

MILLET: A small yellow grain cultivated in Africa, India and China, this staple, an excellent source of potassium and fiber, is versatile enough for use as a cereal or in soups, casseroles and vegetable dishes.

COUSCOUS: This light-colored, partially refined and quick-cooking form of cracked wheat has a taste similar to that of farina. It's used primarily as a side dish with chicken or lamb, or as a base in casseroles.

BARLEY: A good source of potassium and fiber, this rich grain is best in soups or in combination with rice. Whole barley is chewy, while pearl barley is lighter (but it has less nutritional value because its outer grain "coat" has been removed).

RYE: One of the most versatile of the whole grains, rye can be milled in a variety of ways. For example, coarse rye meal is good for making pumpernickel bread, while the grits (cracked rye) are used for cereal. Rye flour is an excellent addition to homemade whole-grain bread. Dark rye is especially rich in fiber, protein, magnesium and potassium.

OATS: Whole-grain oats, or groats, resemble and can be used like long-grain brown rice. Rolled or flattened oats can be combined with milk or water and eaten as is, added to other cold cereals, cooked for a few minutes and eaten as hot oatmeal or used in baking; they are the main ingredient in Muesli, the Swiss breakfast delicacy. For a good dose of soluble fiber, try sprinkling the powdery-fine oat bran over soups, main dishes and desserts. No matter what form they take, oats are a rich source of protein, potassium, magnesium, calcium and phosphorus, along with the B complex and vitamin E.

CORN: This native American grain is most nutritious as whole, stone-ground or enriched cornmeal, which can be used in polenta, corn bread, muffins, corn (hominy) grits and tortillas. Dried corn is soaked in calcium-rich limewater, to get meal for tortillas, making this food an excellent source of the mineral. (Ready-made corn tortillas are available in supermarket freezers. Try new "blue-corn" tortillas for a special treat.) Corn on the cob is a starchy, fibrous vegetable rich in phosphorus and B vitamins. Except for the kind sold in health-food stores, cornflake cereals are generally laced with sugar and sodium; improve on the formula by adding some stone-ground cornmeal, oat and wheat bran and a few fresh berries or nuts. Unsalted, air-popped popcorn, flavored with a trace of herbed olive oil, is an excellent high-fiber, low-calorie snack.

PASTA: On the average, one cup of enriched cooked pasta totals about 200 calories, with a nutritional makeup of protein, carbohydrates, calcium, phosphorus, iron, potassium, magnesium and a number of B vitamins. Pastas made from whole-wheat flours are even richer in nutrients and fiber; the imported Italian varieties have an excellent taste and texture. Those made from gluten or soy flour (often recommended for diabetics) are a superb source of protein. Though called "imitation" by law, pastas made from Jerusalem artichoke flour (ideal for those allergic to wheat, soy or gluten) are virtually indistinguishable from the "real thing."

Meatless tomato (marinara) and light seafood sauces are lowest in calories. In Italy, the pasta itself, not the sauce, is the main event: According to pasta purists, the strands should never be drowned in liquid, but simply coated sparingly.

POTATOES: Ounce for ounce, a potato is no more fattening than an apple or a pear. It's been unjustly maligned, however, perhaps because of french fries or potato chips, which derive 70 percent of their calories from added fat and are altered beyond nutritional recognition! But in its natural form, it's another story: One small (4-ounce) baked potato provides almost half the RDA for vitamin C, and a medium-sized one totals no more than about 90 calories. Sweet potatoes have roughly one-third more calories and a bit less protein, but they also contain more calcium, iron, potassium, niacin and vitamin A than their white counterparts.

Cooking experts advise against using aluminum foil when baking, which results in a *steamed* potato, inferior in texture. Just scrub well, poke a few holes in the top to vent steam and bake in a 450-degree oven for forty-five minutes. A microwave oven can bake a potato in about five minutes.

BEANS AND PEAS (LEGUMES): These are complex carbohydrates married to good-quality protein, plus essential minerals such as phosphorus and potassium. They are the richest sources of protein in the vegetable kingdom. One cup of cooked soybeans has just a little less protein than the same amount of ground beef, without the saturated fat and cholesterol, and with only half the calories.

AMARANTH: This grainlike, seed-bearing plant, a favorite of the early Aztecs, is unusually high in protein, iron and calcium compared to more familiar grains, and contains twice as much fiber as wheat. Amaranth flour can be used in virtually any baked goods, lending them a rich moisture and sweet, nutty flavor.

QUINOA: (pronounced *keen-wa*): This light, highly nutritious grain dates back to the Incas and has been labeled one of the best sources of vegetable protein by the National Academy of Sciences. Found in health-food stores and some supermarkets, it is easy to prepare and can be served as a side dish or main course/casserole just like rice. It also makes a wonderful breakfast cereal.

HIGH FIBER—MACROBIOTIC STYLE

No, Virginia, it's not just brown rice and seaweed! The macrobiotic diet was the subject of controversy during the 1960s, and often justifiably so, when fanatical adherents to some of its principles (who distorted the original concept) became victims of well-publi-

(Continued)

(*Continued*)

cized tragedies. In one instance, former drug addicts, who were most likely in an already nutritionally depleted state, underwent extreme "detoxification" fasts for weeks on end consisting of little more than a few bowlfuls of brown rice a day. Predictably, they soon showed symptoms of serious vitamin and mineral deficiencies, weakness and general malnutrition. In a separate case, several children were placed on too-restricted diets by their overzealous parents in a communal setting: the children were found to have developmental problems, and one even died.

On the other hand, several well-designed studies have shown no adverse nutritional consequences, and decided benefits, from eating a well-balanced, varied macrobiotic diet, the way it was intended to be and in keeping with its basic guidelines.

Hippocrates, the father of Western medicine who so wisely championed fiber, also coined the word "macrobiotic." From the Greek *makro,* meaning long or great, and *bios,* meaning life, the term was first used to describe people who enjoyed good health and longevity. Other classical scientists such as Aristotle, Galen and Herodotus referred to macrobiotics as a life-style and philosophy—including a simple, wholesome diet—that promoted long life and well-being.

In the late nineteenth century, two Japanese educators claimed to have cured themselves of serious illness by following a diet of brown rice, beans, sea vegetables, miso soup and other traditional high-carbohydrate foods. To account for the apparent miracle, they began studying Oriental medicine and philosophy, Judeo-Christian teachings and principles of modern nutrition to integrate these disciplines into a coherent system or way of living. The result was present-day macrobiotics, a diet/ethic that advocates the

(*Continued*)

(*Continued*)

use of unprocessed, unrefined grains, beans and locally grown vegetables as major sources of energy,
and also incorporates mineral-rich seaweeds, soy
products, fermented foods and small amounts of fish.

The typical "macro" meal is rather simple; colorful;
very low in fat, cholesterol and sugar; and high in
fiber, complex carbohydrates and essential nutrients.
A bowl of soup, a dish consisting of one or two whole
grains, some assorted cooked vegetables, a marinated
salad, a bean dish and a small amount of fish (up to
several times a week) make up a customary menu.
The cooked foods are prepared by sautéing, baking,
pressure-cooking, steaming and/or stir-frying to retain
maximum nutritional value. Whole grains are featured
at every meal, and a wide variety of leafy, root and
ground vegetables, mostly cooked or pickled, are recommended daily, along with occasional cooked fruits
(locally grown, if possible). In the macrobiotic
scheme, the whole grains considered most desirable
are brown rice, barley, buckwheat, corn, millet, whole
oats and whole wheat.

One thing that distinguishes this high-fiber diet
from the more Westernized ones is the use of high-
protein soy products, such as tofu and soy milk, to
replace meat and dairy foods. (Rice syrup and barley
malt are used in place of sugar and honey.) In their
natural state, soybeans are difficult to digest because
they contain substances that interfere with our body's
digestive enzymes. However, soybeans that have
been soaked, cooked and fermented are highly digestible and versatile edibles that can be cooked with almost anything and absorb the flavor of surrounding
foods. Tempeh (fermented soy patty) is a rich source
of vitamin B-12 (needed for healthy nerve/muscle
function), which is good news for strict vegetarians,

(*Continued*)

(Continued)

who often have trouble getting enough from their diet.

The macrobiotic diet favors fresh leafy greens in summer and root and ground vegetables during winter months. The greens are good suppliers of vitamin C, calcium and a number of alkaline minerals that counteract excess acidity in the blood. This is considered crucial, since macrobiotic theory holds that an "acid" internal state may make you more susceptible to both major and minor illnesses. Leafy vegetables are also rich in chlorophyll, a valuable source of magnesium. The hardy root vegetables, such as carrots, beets and turnips, and varieties like cabbage and the squash family are thought to be better suited to people living in harsh winter climates.

Other macrobiotic staples include sea vegetables and seaweeds, such as dulse, kelp, nori, kombu and wakame (all available in health-food stores), which are exceedingly rich in iodine; calcium; magnesium; phosphorus; protein; vitamins A, the B complex, C and E; and the trace elements zinc, selenium and chromium. They also have an alkalinizing effect on the blood.

Among the strongest-flavored items on this diet are the fermented foods: sauerkraut, pickles, umeboshi plums, sourdough breads, miso (a soybean paste used mostly in soups and spreads) and tamari soy sauce. Some contain live bacterial cultures that promote the growth of beneficial bacteria and inhibit the trouble-making ones that give rise to intestinal disorders.

If you would like to learn more about macrobiotic cuisine, recipes and philosophy and/or are interested in restaurants that feature "whole food" cooking, contact the East West Foundation, 17 Station Street, Brookline, Massachusetts, 02147.

HOW TO COOK WHOLE GRAINS

Whole grains are without exception simple to prepare and satisfying to eat.

BROWN RICE: Wash 2½ cups rice in a strainer under cold running water to remove any surface starch and dust. Then transfer rice to a pot with a tight-fitting lid and add 4 cups boiling water. Do not stir. Bring to a gentle boil for 2 minutes, cover, turn heat to low and cook for 1 hour. Turn heat up for a few seconds before turning off. Allow rice to sit with the lid on for about 15 minutes before serving.

MILLET: Prepare as for rice, using 2 cups millet to 4½ cups water, and cook for 45 minutes. Millet and rice can be cooked together. Use 1½ cups rice, ½ cup millet; wash and cook using 4 cups of water.

BARLEY: Soak whole barley overnight. Pearled barley may be cooked right away using 1 part barley to 3 or 4 parts rice; add just a bit more water to the normal rice recipe.

BULGUR: Do not wash. Prepare as for rice, using 2 cups bulgur to 2½ cups water and cook for just 20 minutes, or just pour boiling water over and allow to soak for one hour or more.

KASHA: Do not wash. Use whole groats and prepare as for rice, but let the boiling water cool slightly before adding. Bring water to a boil, cover, turn down heat right away and continue cooking for 20 minutes.

WHOLE OATS: These are best cooked overnight on very low heat. Use 1 cup oats to 5 cups water, and make sure your pot is large enough and your flame as *low* as possible. In the morning they will be done and delicious. (You may toast them if you want before cooking.) An alternate approach is to soak them overnight and cook for 2 hours in the morning.

ROLLED OATS: Do not wash. Prepare as for rice, using 1 cup oats to 2 cups water. Cook for 25 minutes.

STEEL-CUT OATS: Do not wash. Prepare as for rice, using 1 cup oats to 3 cups water.

Vary the flavor of grains by using vegetable stock instead of water, adding fresh herbs or toasted nuts or seeds, toasting the grains in a small amount of fragrant cold-pressed olive or sesame oil and/or placing some mineral-rich kombu seaweed in the pot before cooking.

SAMPLE MENUS

Recipes are provided for all dishes marked with an asterisk (*). To find recipes that appear in other sections, consult the Index at the back of this book.

Beverages for all meals: herbal tea, black coffee, instant grain coffee (e.g., Caffix), skim milk, soy milk, seltzer, plain or sparkling mineral water, fresh vegetable juices or filtered tap water.

DAY 1:

Breakfast

Muesli (Swiss cold oat cereal): ½ cup uncooked rolled oats with ⅓ cup mixed sliced banana and apple, 1 tablespoon chopped almonds (optional) and ½ cup skim or soy milk. For added fiber in this and all morning cereals (and lunch and dinner entrees or desserts), top with 1 to 2 tablespoons each oat and wheat bran.

Lunch

1 cup Hearty Lentil Soup*

1 whole-wheat pita pocket stuffed with 1–2 ounces low-fat (1 percent) cottage cheese, chopped fresh scallions, grated carrot, romaine leaves, raw broccoli, shredded cabbage (or any other fresh herb/vegetable combo)

Dinner

Festive Vegetable Stir-Fry with Oriental Brown Rice*

Tossed escarole and bell pepper salad with yogurt relish (plain low- or nonfat yogurt mixed with lemon juice and horseradish to taste)

½ cup High-Fiber Fresh Fruit Compote*

Snacks

1 apple

1 tablespoon sunflower seeds

1 cup air-popped popcorn with fresh chopped herbs and dash of olive oil

DAY 2:

Breakfast

1 or 2 Super Grain Pancakes* topped with cinnamon or ¼ cup Low-Cal Fresh Strawberry Syrup*

Lunch

Pasta salad, such as cold pasta primavera salad (4 ounces whole-wheat or semolina pasta tossed with 1 teaspoon olive oil, fresh tomatoes, garlic, black olives, capers, parsley)

Chilled unpeeled pear slices with ¾ cup plain low- or nonfat yogurt or vanilla kefir, sprinkled with 1 tablespoon each wheat and oat bran

Dinner

4 ounces Chicken in Wine and Mushroom Sauce* *or* Savory Oven-Grilled Tofu*

½ cup each chopped steamed broccoli and carrots with fresh herbs and toasted sesame seeds

Tossed romaine and fresh cabbage salad with apple slices, dressed with 1 teaspoon each soy oil and lemon juice

Snacks

3–4 chestnuts

Oat Bran Muffin* with 1 cup skim milk

1 cup carrot and celery juice

DAY 3:

Breakfast

½ cup Homemade Crunchy Granola* with ½ cup each skim or soy milk, fresh berries or banana slices

Lunch

Spicy Middle Eastern Hummus (chickpea spread)* with raw veggies on whole-wheat pita bread *or* Open-Faced Cheese Sandwich*

Orange-red leaf salad (orange slices over red leaf lettuce, topped with grated cabbage and carrots)

Dinner

Baked Stuffed Acorn Squash* with millet or brown rice *or* Baked Broccoli- or Zucchini-Cheese Casserole (½ cup chopped broccoli or zucchini, partially steamed, topped with a mixture of grated part-skim cheese or low-fat cottage cheese, chopped onion, fresh Italian parsley, ground pepper, oregano, basil and whole-wheat bread crumbs [optional]. Bake for 4–5 minutes or until cheese melts.)

Steamed cauliflower and bok choy (Chinese cabbage) with lemon juice

Salad of chives, shredded romaine, radish and carrot with 1 tablespoon any fruit vinegar

Snacks

2 brown rice cakes with 1 teaspoon pureed fresh fruit, fruit conserves or apple butter

DAY 4:

Breakfast

High-Fiber Omelet (made with 1 egg and 1 egg white, chopped raw vegetables, 1 teaspoon grated Parmesan cheese and 1 tablespoon each wheat and oat bran) *or* Scrambled Tofu Omelet (sauté any favorite chopped vegetables and herbs in a small amount of olive oil for 2–3 minutes; add 3 ounces diced or crumbled tofu and continue sautéing for 3–4 more minutes).

1 whole-grain English muffin

Lunch

Homemade Couscous Salad* *or* a large spinach salad with mushrooms, beets, tomatoes and sprouts

½ cantaloupe, topped with plain low- or nonfat yogurt

Dinner

1 Salmon-Stuffed Potato*

½ cup thinly sliced zucchini sautéed in 1 teaspoon olive oil with water chestnuts and scallions

Chicory salad with lemon juice and chopped fresh dill

1 medium pear or apple, unpeeled

Snacks

2 Wasa crackers with ½ teaspoon sesame butter

½ cup skim milk

DAY 5:

Breakfast

½ cup oatmeal, Wheatena, cream of rye or Hot Millet Breakfast Cereal (½ cup cooked millet with raisins) with cinnamon, fresh berries and sunflower seeds *or* 1 Oat Bran Muffin* with ½ teaspoon apple butter

1 cup skim or soy milk *or* ¾ cup plain low- or nonfat yogurt

1 orange or half grapefruit

Lunch

1 cup bouillon *or* ½ cup black bean soup

No-Ham Burger* with lettuce, tomato, carrots and sprouts on whole-wheat roll

1 medium apple

Dinner

Pasta Shells with Broccoli and Parmesan*

Tossed dandelion, curly lettuce and tomato salad with tarragon vinegar

½ cup fresh fruit salad with ½ cup plain low- or nonfat yogurt

Snacks

2 corn tostadas with grated carrot

DAY 6:

Breakfast

½ cup Nutri-Grain Corn, Müeslix, Shredded Wheat 'n Bran, Crispy Brown Rice or amaranth cereal (the last two are available in health-food stores) with ½ cup skim or soy milk

½ cup apple, orange and banana fruit salad

Lunch

½ cup Kasha with Mushrooms 'n' Onions* *or* 1 cup assorted steamed or raw vegetables with lemon juice

1 slice multigrain bread or whole-wheat pita pocket with 1 ounce low-fat cheese (e.g. part-skim Jarlsberg, mozzarella or farmer cheese)

½ cup green grapes with 1 cup plain low- or nonfat yogurt

Dinner

½ cup Paella Paradise* *or* ½ cup red beans, with rice (sauté canned or cooked beans with garlic, onion and any chopped vegetables and 1 teaspoon olive oil before adding to cooked rice).

Steamed asparagus spears with 1 teaspoon low-cal mayonnaise

Half papaya filled with strawberries and kiwis

Red, white and green salad: watercress, red pepper

and cauliflower with 1 teaspoon each olive oil and tarragon vinegar

Snacks

2 oatcakes or oat crackers (available at gourmet and health-food stores) with 1–2 tablespoons Miso Scallion Spread* (delicious!)

DAY 7:

Breakfast

1 slice Fiber-Rich French Toast*

½ grapefruit

Lunch

1 Rice-Stuffed Cabbage Roll* *or* 1 serving Curried Rice Salad*

Carrot-Raisin Salad (grated carrots and 2 tablespoons raisins sprinkled with lemon) with 2 ounces low-fat (1 percent) cottage cheese

Dinner

1 cup Vegetarian Chili with Rice* *or* 1 cup Luscious Lentil Stew*

Cucumber and onion salad with Tofu-Sesame Dressing*

Snacks

1 Oat Bran Muffin* with 1 teaspoon pureed fresh fruit or fruit conserves

¾ cup plain low- or nonfat yogurt (with cinnamon or vanilla for flavoring)

▪

FIVE EASY PIECES

Satisfying, nutritious, portable lunch/dinner alternatives that you can prepare with a minimum of fuss or
effort. Each makes one individual portion.

1. *Raw vegetables with onion-yogurt dip*
   Add ½ contents of instant onion soup mix to 1 cup
   low-fat yogurt. Use as flavorful dip for celery, radishes, green or red pepper slices, scallions and raw
   cauliflower/broccoli florets.

2. *Quick rice and bean salad plus instant oat broth*
   Mix ½ cup each leftover (preferably brown) rice
   and cooked beans (any kind) with grated carrots,
   chopped scallions, celery and green pepper (or any
   vegetable combo) and 1 tablespoon plain yogurt on
   low-cal mayonnaise. Serve cold. For broth, dissolve ½ vegetable broth cube in cup of hot water.
   Add 3 tablespoons oat bran and allow to stand for
   5 minutes. A warm, hearty pick-me-up!

3. *Whole-grain pita pocket*
   Add chili "salsa" and fresh or dried herbs to ½ cup
   low-fat (1 percent) cottage cheese to taste. Pack
   into whole-grain pita bread with fresh sprouts,
   shredded cabbage, tomatoes and onion slices.

4. *Sprout sandwich*
   Garnish whole-grain bread liberally with Dijon
   mustard, then layer with sliced cucumbers, tomatoes, and two ounces low-fat cheese (optional)
   topped with bran and mixed sprouts.

5. *Instant miso soup*
   Add instant noodles to 1 cup freshly boiled water,
   mix in contents of Miso-Cup (instant soup available in health-food stores), and garnish with a few

sprigs of fresh spinach or watercress, or chopped scallions. Eat with high-fiber crackers or whole-grain bread topped with 1 teaspoon nut butter.

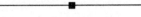

RECIPES

Hearty lentil soup   *1st Day Lunch*

1 cup dry lentils
3 cups water
1 cup diced carrots
¾ cups chopped celery
½ cup chopped broccoli
¾ cup chopped onion
1 teaspoon salt *or* 1½ tablespoons tamari (soy) sauce
Handful of chopped parsley
1 tablespoon olive oil

Bring lentils to a boil. Reduce heat, add remaining ingredients and simmer 30–35 minutes. *Serves 8.*

Festive vegetable stir-fry with oriental brown rice   *1st Day Dinner*

1½ tablespoons peanut oil
1 clove garlic, minced
½ cup each, sliced: broccoli
     carrrots
     cauliflower
     onion
     bok choy (or celery)
     cabbage
1 tablespoon water
1½ teaspoons sesame oil
½ cup sliced mushrooms
2 cups cooked brown rice
1½ teaspoons natural soy (shoyu) sauce

Heat peanut oil. Add onions and garlic. Sauté until golden.
Add sliced vegetables and stir-fry. Add water when oil dries
out. Stir 4 minutes, cover and remove from heat. Heat sesame
oil and add sliced mushrooms. Stir 3 minutes. Mix in cooked
brown rice and soy sauce. Top with sautéed vegetables.
Serves 4.

High-fiber fresh fruit compote   1st Day Dinner

½ cup pineapple slices
¼ cup apple juice
1 each, diced (unpeeled): apple
                           pear
                           peach
                           apricot

Blend pineapple and apple juice at high speed. Pour over
½ cup servings of diced fruit. *Serves 4.*

Super grain pancakes   2nd Day Breakfast

Pancake Mix:

2 cups whole-wheat flour
1 cup soy flour
1 cup buckwheat flour
1 cup rolled oats
½ cup whole cornmeal
1 cup wheat germ
¼ cup powdered lecithin

Combine mix ingredients and store in a tightly closed container.

Pancakes:

2 egg whites
1 cup skim or soy milk
1 cup pancake mix
2 tablespoons safflower or vegetable oil

½ teaspoon baking powder
1 tablespoon honey

Beat egg whites with milk and slowly add pancake mix. Add remaining ingredients, stirring until well mixed. Cook on hot oiled griddle. Turn when the edges begin to get firm. *Serves 3 (makes 6–8 pancakes).*

Low-cal fresh strawberry syrup   *2nd Day Breakfast*

¼ cup maple syrup
1 cup apple juice
2 teaspoons cornstarch
Pinch of salt
½ cup sliced fresh strawberries

Mix together maple syrup, apple juice, cornstarch and salt. Bring to a boil over medium heat, stirring constantly until thick. Remove from heat and stir in sliced strawberries. Serve warm over pancakes.

Chicken in wine and mushroom sauce   *2nd Day Dinner*

½ teaspoon each, salt and pepper
1½ teaspoons whole-wheat flour
1 pound chicken breasts, halved
1 tablespoon olive oil
1 small onion, chopped
¼ cup white wine
1 teaspoon tomato paste
¼ cup chicken stock or bouillon
¼ cup wine vinegar
1 clove garlic, minced
2 teaspoons chopped parsley
¼ cup sliced mushrooms

Combine salt, pepper and flour. Rub on chicken. Heat olive oil in a skillet. Add onion and sauté 4 minutes, stirring. Add the chicken and brown lightly. Add wine and cook over medium-high heat for 4 minutes. Combine tomato paste and stock and add to chicken, stirring. Reduce heat to medium and cook 40 minutes, or until chicken is tender.

Bring wine vinegar to a boil and cook 2 minutes on high heat. Add garlic, parsley, mushrooms and simmer for a minute. Pour over the chicken and serve. *Serves 4.*

Savory oven-grilled tofu   2nd Day Dinner

12 ounces cake "firm" tofu
1 teaspoon dark sesame oil
2 teaspoons arrowroot
¾ cup water
¼ cup tamari (soy) sauce
1 teaspoon finely grated ginger
1 scallion, chopped

Preheat oven to 450 degrees. Slice tofu into ½ inch "cutlets." Oil broiler pan or cookie sheet with sesame oil and add tofu. Bake in oven 15–20 minutes or until lightly browned.

Meanwhile, dissolve arrowroot in cold water and heat mixture to a boil in a small saucepan; add tamari, grated ginger, and scallion, simmering gently to a thick consistency. Pour sauce over tofu "cutlets" and serve. *Serves 2–3.*

Oat bran muffins   2nd Day Snack

¼ cup oat bran
1 cup oat flour
¼ cup brown rice flour

4 teaspoons Arrowroot
  Baking Powder*
½ teaspoon salt
1 cup skim or soy milk
3 tablespoons rice syrup or
  barley malt (sweetener)
2 tablespoons safflower oil
3 tablespoons chopped
  walnuts
¼ cup chopped dates
  (optional)

Preheat oven to 400 degrees. Combine bran, flour, baking powder and salt. Mix soy milk, sweetener and oil together, then stir into flour 1 minute until moistened. Add walnuts and dates. Spoon into well-greased muffin pan. Bake for 20–25 minutes until browned. *Serves 4.*

* *Arrowroot Baking Powder:* Combine ⅓ cup baking soda, ⅔ cup cream of tartar and ⅔ cup arrowroot. Mix well. Store in airtight container. (1 teaspoon baking powder = 1½ teaspoons arrowroot baking powder.)

Homemade crunchy granola　　　　　*3rd Day Breakfast*

2½ cups rolled oats
¼ cup sesame seeds
⅓ cup sunflower seeds
½ cup soy grits (optional)
1 teaspoon cinnamon
1 teaspoon vanilla
½ cup rice flour
½ cup nonfat dry milk or
  powdered soy milk
½ cup unsweetened
  coconut, grated
3 tablespoons undiluted
  apple juice concentrate,
  thawed

Preheat oven to 275 degrees. Combine ingredients. Put mixture on large flat nonstick pan. Spread evenly into a thin layer. Bake for 35–45 minutes until mixture is dry. Crumble to desired consistency. Store in covered container. (Refrigerates well.) *Serves 8.*

Spicy Middle Eastern hummus   3rd Day Lunch

3 cups cooked* or canned, drained chickpeas
½ cup chickpea cooking water or unsalted broth
3 tablespoons sesame butter or tahini
Juice of 1½ lemons
1 tablespoon olive oil
2 scallions, chopped
¼ teaspoon paprika
3 cloves garlic, finely chopped
⅔ cup chopped parsley
1 teaspoon sea salt

In food processor or blender combine all ingredients and blend until fairly smooth. *Serves 8.*

Open-faced cheese sandwich   3rd Day Lunch

Olive oil
Chopped fresh or dried oregano
Basil
2 slices whole-wheat or rye bread, toasted
1½ ounces skim mozzarella cheese, sliced thin
Sliced tomato

* *Cooking Instructions for Chickpeas:* Wash 1½ cups chickpeas; clean out stones. Soak overnight. In the morning drain and add 5 cups fresh water. Bring to a boil, then lower heat and simmer until soft (about 1 hour and 15 minutes)—best done on a weekend! Drain, reserving ½ cup liquid for hummus. For a much quicker recipe, use canned chickpeas, of course.

Combine oil and herbs. Brush on top of toast and cheese. Place 2–3 tomato slices on top of cheese. Place open-faced sandwiches in broiler. It takes about 2 minutes for cheese to melt. Don't walk away from broiler! *Serves 2.*

Baked stuffed acorn squash   *3rd Day Dinner*

1 medium-sized acorn squash
½ cup cooked millet or brown rice
¼ cup cooked or canned, drained peas
¼ cup cooked or canned, drained mushrooms
⅓ cup grated onions
1 medium carrot, diced
½ teaspoon coriander
1 teaspoon basil
½ teaspoon salt
1½ tablespoons olive oil

Preheat oven to 400 degrees. Slice squash lengthwise, remove seeds and place face-down in shallow baking pan with a little water. Bake for approximately 30 minutes or until soft. Combine remaining ingredients, mix well and fill squash. Continue heating for 3–5 minutes. *Serves 2.*

Homemade couscous salad   *4th Day Lunch*

½ cup couscous
1½ cups water
1 stalk celery, diced
1 small carrot, diced
1 small onion, diced
½ teaspoon tarragon
Dash turmeric
½ teaspoon salt
1 tablespoon olive oil

Bring couscous to a boil, lower flame and simmer. Add diced vegetables, herbs, salt and oil. Cover and cook until water is absorbed (about 15 minutes). Chill. (Refrigerates well.) *Serves 4 to 6.*

Salmon-stuffed potatoes   *4th Day Dinner*

4 potatoes
½ cup low-fat buttermilk
½ cup water-packed salmon
Paprika to taste
½ teaspoon sage
Chopped parsley and scallions to taste

Bake potatoes at 425 degrees for 55 minutes. Cut potatoes in half and scoop out pulp. Mash pulp, then blend in buttermilk until mashed potato consistency is reached. Flake salmon with fork and stir into mashed potato. Restuff potato shells, and sprinkle with paprika and remaining herbs and spices. *Serves 4.*

No-ham burgers   *5th Day Lunch*

2 cups cooked or canned, drained soybeans
½ cup grated, drained carrots
½ cup thinly sliced celery
½ cup finely chopped cooked onion
3 tablespoons olive or sesame oil
1 tablespoon chopped fresh or dried parsley
2 tablespoons tamari (soy) sauce
½ teaspoon salt
¼ teaspoon cumin
2 tablespoons arrowroot flour

Preheat oven to 375–400 degrees. Combine and grind up ingredients in blender or food processor; mix well. The consistency should be almost like that of applesauce, but slightly coarser. Form into patties by hand, or use ice cream scoop and flatten to about ⅓ to ½ inch thickness and 3 inches diameter. Lightly oil a flat baking pan; place patties in pan. Bake for about 35 minutes or until golden brown. Burgers may be turned over midway, but it's not necessary. *Yields approximately 8–10 burgers. Refrigerates or freezes well.*

Pasta shells with broccoli and parmesan   5th Day Dinner

8 ounces pasta shells from any whole grain
2 teaspoons olive oil
1 clove garlic, minced
2 cups chopped broccoli
½ teaspoon oregano
½ teaspoon basil
Pinch of salt
2 tablespoons grated Parmesan

Cook pasta and drain. Heat oil in skillet and sauté garlic and broccoli 5 minutes. Add water if oil dries. Add seasonings, stirring another minute. Add to pasta shells and sprinkle Parmesan on top. *Serves 4.*

Kasha with mushrooms 'n' onions   6th Day Lunch

¾ cup kasha
1½ cups water
1 large onion, chopped
½ cup sliced mushrooms
¾ teaspoon salt
2 tablespoons sesame oil
1 tablespoon sesame seeds

Bring kasha to a boil and cook for 10–12 minutes or until fluffy. In a skillet or frying pan sauté onion with remaining

ingredients. Mix with kasha and serve. (Refrigerates well.)
Serves 3.

Paella paradise   *6th Day Dinner*

½ cup olive oil
1 large onion, chopped
1 cup cooked long-grain
   brown rice
2 cloves garlic, finely
   chopped
1 cup quartered tomatoes
2 saffron strands
1 quart broth or water
½ teaspoon sage
¼ teaspoon marjoram
¼ teaspoon paprika
Dash of pepper
½ pound shelled, deveined
   shrimp
1 sweet red pepper
1 cup cauliflower
½ cup cooked or canned
   kidney beans
1 cup sliced snow peas

Heat oil in flameproof casserole. Add onion and cook until
transparent. Add rice and garlic and fry for 2 minutes, stirring
often. Add tomatoes, saffron, broth and seasonings and bring
to a boil. Reduce heat and simmer for 15 minutes. Cut shrimp
into bite-sized pieces. Halve the pepper and cut into 1-inch
pieces. Cut cauliflower into pieces. Drain the beans. Add all
ingredients to the pan along with snow peas and mix lightly.
Cover and cook for 15 minutes or until rice is tender and
liquid is absorbed. When finished fluff with a fork. *Serves 4.*

Miso scallion spread   6th Day Snack

1 cup "light" yellow or white miso (found in health-food
  stores or Oriental groceries)
1 scallion, chopped
2 tablespoons oat flour
½ cup warm water
2 tablespoons chopped toasted sunflower seeds (optional)

Blend ingredients thoroughly, and refrigerate for 1 hour before serving. Spread lightly on high-fiber wheat or rye thins
or brown-rice crackers.

Fiber-rich french toast   7th Day Breakfast

1 egg
1 tablespoon skim milk
2 slices whole-grain bread
2 teaspoons soy oil
¼ teaspoon cinnamon

Beat egg and milk together. Dip bread in the mixture. Cook
on an oiled skillet until brown on one side. Turn, sprinkle
with cinnamon and brown other side. Serve with fruit conserves or a little maple syrup. *Serves 2.*

Rice-stuffed cabbage rolls   7th Day Lunch

4 large cabbage leaves
⅓ cup each: chopped carrot, zucchini, broccoli, onion
⅓ cup green peas
1½ cups cooked brown rice
2 tablespoons safflower oil
½ teaspoon sea salt
1 tablespoon tamari (soy) sauce
½ tablespoon curry powder
1 tablespoon dried or chopped fresh parsley

Steam vegetables in stainless steel steamer basket for approximately 7–10 minutes, or until tender. Set cabbage leaves aside. Combine chopped vegetables with remaining ingredients and mix well. Place ¼ of mixture on the center of each cooked cabbage leaf and roll. *Serves 2.*

Curried rice salad 7th Day Lunch

1 pound tofu, diced
1 onion, minced
2½ cups cooked, chilled brown rice
2 tablespoons minced parsley
Lettuce
1 celery stalk
2 tomatoes, cut into wedges

Combine tofu, onion, rice and parsley. Serve on lettuce and garnish with celery and tomato.

Dressing:
4 tablespoons peanut oil
1 teaspoon curry powder
2 tablespoons lemon juice
1 clove garlic, minced
1 tablespoon tamari (soy) sauce

Mix and pour over salad.

Serves 8.

Vegetarian chili with rice 7th Day Dinner

½ pound dry kidney beans
6 cups water
2½ to 3 cups cooked brown rice
2 onions, chopped
4 celery stalks, chopped
1 zucchini squash, sliced
2 cloves garlic, minced

1 tablespoon olive oil
½ pound tomatoes, cut
2 tablespoons chopped scallion
½ teaspoon chili powder
½ teaspoon oregano

Soak beans overnight in water. Prepare rice; cook beans ¾ hour on low heat. Sauté onions, celery, zucchini and garlic in oil. Add to beans. Add tomatoes, scallion and seasonings. Cook until vegetables are done. Serve over rice. *Serves 6.*

Luscious lentil stew   *7th Day Dinner*

3 cups water
Dash olive oil (cold-pressed)
½ cup finely diced celery
½ cup chopped onion
½ cup lentils, washed
2 cups chopped fresh tomato
½ cup shredded carrots
½ teaspoon rosemary
2 cloves garlic, chopped

Bring water, oil, celery, onion and lentils to a boil. Simmer 20 minutes. Combine remaining ingredients, add to lentils. Simmer together for 45 minutes. Add salt and pepper to taste. *Serves 4.*

Tofu-sesame dressing   *7th Day Dinner*

2 ounces tofu (¼ of an 8-ounce square), crumbled
1 tablespoon sesame butter (tahini)
1 teaspoon dark sesame oil
2 tablespoons brown rice vinegar
¼ cup water
Dash of grated fresh ginger

Blend all ingredients well. *Makes about ½ cup.*

5

DIET TYPE 2

The Modified Protein-Plus Diet

You can find it everywhere—in skin and bone, cartilage and muscle, blood and lymph, nerves, hair, nails and teeth; not a single cell in your body can exist without it, and it must be constantly replenished. The major component in enzymes and hormones, it's the most active, versatile player in your internal universe. It repairs injured and worn-out tissues, builds new ones, ushers nutrients in and out of cells. It's the raw material from which lifesaving antibodies, the guardians of your immune system, are formed. Its components, known as amino acids, are necessary for vitamins and minerals to be put to proper use.

No wonder protein carries such clout. To most of us, it's synonymous with health, vitality and longevity. And, until recently, the high-protein diet was considered the best way to lose weight. If you wanted to shed 5 or even 10 or 20 pounds fairly fast—say, in time for your best friend's wedding or an important job interview—you'd choose from diets with household names like Atkins, Stillman or Scarsdale to see you through.

They all worked in much the same way. The simple, easy-to-prepare meals allowed generous, even "unlimited" helpings of steak, chicken, cheese and burgers without the bun; they were far stingier with potatoes, pasta, bread and other carbohydrates (which everyone labeled too fattening)—and the results were often *sensational*. The pounds would fall away quickly, without much effort. The diets probably resembled the way you ate already, so you didn't have to significantly change your mealtime habits. The familiar, no-frill foods were readily available, easy to find at restaurants, take-out counters and weekend dinner parties. They were the stick-to-the-ribs kind, so you never felt too deprived. The formula seemed foolproof: What more could a dieter ask?

In our quest for the quick fix, however, we overlooked some sobering facts. For one thing, most of the discarded pounds were in the form of water; excess protein causes our bodies to excrete it at a faster rate. (The body's tissues release fluids to dilute the toxic byproducts of protein and fat metabolism, called "ketones." Thirst and dehydration are common results.) The weight loss was strictly temporary, too; by week two or three, we would be in a holding pattern. We would also find ourselves more tired and lethargic than we'd ever been, and even bothered by occasional nausea, headaches or diarrhea.

What could possibly be wrong with a diet based on our body's primary nutrient? The biggest problem is not so much the presence of protein but rather the *shortage of carbohydrates*. These are our most direct and efficient source of energy, available to cells immediately or stored for long-term use. Designed as ready-made fuel, carbohydrates are converted simply into glucose ("cell food") plus the waste materials carbon dioxide and water, which the body easily eliminates. When we don't get enough carbohydrates from our diet, however, the body is forced to rely on protein instead for its energy. But protein's chief purpose is to build and repair body tissues; as an energy source, it's highly inefficient since it leaves behind undesirable residues, and these put extra stress on the kidneys, liver and colon.

A protein-based diet has many advantages, particularly when you're trying to lose those first extra pounds, but be sure you don't overlook carbohydrates. Without an adequate amount, protein can't do its job effectively—with possible harmful consequences. As a nation, we're already getting far more protein than we need; a surplus has been linked to shorter life expectancy, increased risk of cancer and heart disease, osteoporosis and, yes, obesity.

For all their effectiveness in a short-term diet, animal proteins—meat, poultry, dairy foods, eggs—come too often with fatty strings attached. For example, 80 percent of the calories from a sirloin steak are from saturated fat, and only 15 percent are from protein.

One patient of mine had been on a high-protein regimen supervised by a noted diet program. She was allowed a generous dose of animal protein, with liberal quantities of eggs and fatty meats, but her daily quota of vegetables had been limited to two small green salads. Initially, she lost weight at a steady, rapid pace—almost seven pounds in the first week alone—but soon after, she leveled off and started complaining of fatigue and sluggishness. She became concerned that for some quick results she might pay a steep long-term price. Sure enough, a blood test confirmed her worst fears. Her cholesterol had soared nearly 200 points since she'd started the high-protein diet!

Keep in mind that "high" is the key word here: Protein-rich meals are wonderful, necessary, very nutritious and an ideal foundation for effective weight loss. You'll find plenty of these foods on the menu for this Diet Type—but not an excessive amount, way out of proportion to the essential carbohydrates. Remember, trouble arises only when a diet is too lopsided in favor of protein foods—and the not-so-healthy kinds at that.

ON THE PLUS SIDE

What's *good* about protein? How can it be part of a successful diet strategy? When calories are carefully controlled, predominantly protein meals can eliminate more unwanted pounds in a given period than those rich in carbohydrates. This is true especially for people who tend to be "carbohydrate cravers." They binge on bread and starchy sweets, but eat less when presented with a protein meal. A recent study at the Dartmouth Medical School showed that dieters who ate a higher proportion of proteins to carbohydrates lost an average of 11 pounds, compared to 8 in a contrasting group. The researchers also found only minor differences in the blood-fat levels of the two groups; those on the protein plan did not show much of an increase in either their cholesterol or triglycerides when they restricted their total intake to about 1,000 low-fat and well-varied calories a day.

There are other pluses: Because the body digests it rather slowly, protein is an effective appetite-appeaser. Protein foods are easy to buy and plan meals around, to socialize and travel with, especially on the business circuit; after all, they're the well-liked mainstays of American cuisine.

One medical condition that specifically benefits from protein nutrition is a chronic respiratory problem found in people with severe emphysema or lung fibrosis. Those with serious pulmonary disease may accumulate toxic levels of carbon dioxide in their bodies, a condition that can be aggravated by a diet too high in carbohydrates. People who breathe normally have no trouble getting rid of the surplus carbon dioxide. A protein-rich, low-carbohydrate regimen, however, can help ease symptoms such as shortness of breath. In a recent study at the University of Wales College of Medicine, a protein-dominant diet improved the general well-being and breathing capacity of patients with chronic respiratory failure.

Overweight women are more likely than men to be carbohydrate cravers. A start-up protein plan can help them lose weight by breaking their addictive habits. Some people with hypoglycemia respond well to a predominantly protein diet, since it releases sugar into the bloodstream gradually. Hypoglycemics thrive on complex carbohydrates, which keep blood-sugar levels relatively stable, too. Some people with common allergies to grains, or who experience more-than-usual gas or bloating after eating high-carbohydrate meals, may benefit from a protein-centered diet, too, since it downplays breads and cereals, the source of their problem. They simply tolerate proteins better and find them more digestible. In fact, certain carbohydrate foods contain enzymes that act as powerful digestion inhibitors (see Diet Type 1).

MODERATION IS EVERYTHING

Think of protein as a powerhouse; a little goes a very long way. In fact, this wonder nutrient should make up no more than 10 to 15 percent of your daily calories. This means simply that any *high*-protein diet will definitely be drastic and imbalanced!

According to the latest government statistics, infants and children on average consume about twice the Recommended Dietary Allowance (RDA) for protein. The average middle-aged man takes in 60 percent more than the recommended level, and the average middle-aged woman about 25 percent more. And experts challenge the RDAs themselves as being too high, because in many countries that show a lower incidence of degenerative diseases, protein consumption is half or even a third of what it is in the United States. We already know that protein needs diminish with age. Relative to their weight, babies require almost three times as much as adults. Unfortunately, too many of us are eating as if we were still in infancy!

On the other hand, nutritional surveys show that many elderly patients, particularly those with digestive diseases or dental problems or whose general weakness prevents them from shopping or cooking, rely too heavily on refined foods like white bread and quick-cooking rice, ultimately courting protein malnutrition.

What are some of the consequences of *excess?* Besides being too often teamed with saturated fat and cholesterol, animal protein leaves nitrogen residues in the bloodstream, which your kidneys are forced to flush away. This constant cleanup job puts extra stress on these natural filters, and they may not be designed to handle the work load. After all, the body's organs evolved at a time when humans were hunter-gatherers who subsisted largely on nuts, seeds and plants, only occasionally eating protein-rich wild game. So the kidney probably needs plenty of rest between protein "feasts."

In fact, high-protein diets are associated with kidney damage in laboratory animals. The same pattern applies to humans, which means that anyone with an already existing kidney-related disorder should be particularly careful about his or her protein intake.

The only reason high-protein diets always require drinking at least eight to ten glasses of water a day is to help "irrigate" the kidneys and rid them of accumulated toxins— not a pretty picture! Because the nitrogen wastes from protein are acidic, the body draws on its alkaline minerals such as calcium, magnesium and zinc to neutralize them. As a result, these vital nutrients are excreted along with the unwanted residues. And that can put you in a state called "negative mineral balance": You lose more minerals than you're taking in. The more protein you consume, the more calcium may wind up in your urine and the less in your bones.

A report by the University of Wisconsin's Department of Nutritional Sciences concludes that substantial mineral loss could result after a decade or so of eating too much protein, which may heighten the risk of osteoporosis, or weak, fracture-prone bones. Not surprisingly, among ten population groups examined in one recent study, those who ate the most protein, such as Americans and New Zealanders, showed the highest rate of hip fracture, one index of osteoporosis. These same groups also consumed the most calcium!

In the U.S., the subspecialty of orthopedics is today largely

PROTEIN FOODS:
A NEW ANGLE ON CHOLESTEROL

Some little-known and still-preliminary research suggests that the *way* certain fatty protein foods are prepared influences cholesterol's destructive impact on the body. This finding may be of particular concern to those of us who do need to monitor our food intake with special care. Early in this century, the Indian working-class immigrants of London showed a dramatically higher rate of heart disease than the rest of the city's population. Trying to solve the puzzle, physicians discovered that the Indians as a rule prepared much of their food using *ghee,* butter that has been clarified to remove its creamy film. When the butter was subsequently heated to very high temperatures for frying, its cholesterol became highly oxidized, possibly making it more prone to damage delicate arterial membranes. Some studies have shown that fried or hard-boiled (well-cooked) eggs produce atherosclerosis most quickly in rabbits—at ten to fourteen times the normal rate—while raw or soft-boiled eggs speed up the process by only three or four times. Scrambled eggs yield an intermediate six- or sevenfold atherosclerosis increase. (Since rabbits don't ordinarily eat cholesterol-containing food, more experiments are now under way to confirm this controversial theory.)

Foods that contain potentially worrisome amounts of oxidized cholesterol include beef tallow (used for frying, especially in fast-food restaurants) as well as charbroiled meats and powdered dry milk, which is prepared via a process of heating and dehydration. Exposure to air for long periods may also oxidize cho-

(Continued)

(Continued)

lesterol. For example, processed cheeses that are in contact with oxygen for a long time during their manufacture and then are stored at room temperature may contain significant quantities of toxic cholesterol derivatives.

For those who are cholesterol-sensitive or otherwise at risk of coronary disease, I suggest a low-saturated-fat diet and sparing use of any cholesterol-rich staples, such as butter and eggs, in as unoxidized—gently cooked or "soft"—a form as possible. Thus, creamy or whipped tub butter may be preferable to the stick kind, spread as is or heated just to the melting point when used in cooking or baking; soft-boiled, poached, sunny-side up or "over easy" eggs with liquid yolks are possibly more desirable than hard-boiled, powdered or scrambled eggs.

devoted to high-tech hip replacement—virtually always the consequence of bone erosion due to osteoporosis in the elderly. But in the otherwise advanced medical system of Japan, a country which used to rely heavily on a traditional diet of rice, vegetables and sparing amounts of fish, with practically *no* calcium-rich dairy products, orthopedics had always lagged behind other medical subspecialties. Today, however, with the importing of large amounts of beef and new "gourmet" products such as cheese and ice cream, orthopedics is beginning to assume a new importance as the rate of osteoporosis in Japan begins to keep stride with that of other advanced countries.

What is crucial is the *kind* of protein you overeat. Studies have shown that simply feeding laboratory animals large amounts of casein, a milk protein, without *any* accompanying fat can increase their blood cholesterol. However, the same amount of soy protein, derived from plants, may have just the opposite effect.

Cancer enters the picture, too. The widely publicized

Diet, Nutrition and Cancer report from the National Academy of Sciences observed that high animal-protein intake may be associated with an increased risk of malignancies at certain sites, including the breast, endometrium, colon, rectum, pancreas and kidney. While nutritionists have attributed the harmful effects of excess protein to the "bad company" it keeps—namely fats—animal studies show that *protein by itself* can be a troublemaker. Colin Campbell, a cancer researcher at Cornell University and an author of the NAS report, explains that animal protein promotes cancer more dramatically than does fat: While fatty diets definitely stimulate tumors, animals fed extra doses of casein and exposed to a known carcinogen develop even more tumorous growths. Apparently, fats and protein trigger malignancy in different ways, and their effects may reinforce each other.

Too much of the wrong protein can also elevate uric acid levels, increasing the risk of gout. (Gout occurs when the acid reaches extremely high concentration in the blood and the spaces between joints, resulting in pain and inflammation.) Most animal proteins and organ meats contain substances called purines, which are linked to both gout and uric acid stones.

Still another concern about protein foods is that many of them tend to concentrate environmental pollutants. The higher up you go in the food chain—and animals top the list—the greater the accumulation of DDT and other pesticide residues. In addition, meats often contain hormones, antibiotics, tranquilizers, enzymes and/or dyes that have been injected directly into animals or added to their feed.

As if this weren't enough, always favoring animal protein may also make you fat. A spartan 2-ounce portion of meat, chicken or fish is all you need to get more than a third of your daily allowance for protein, and the rest of your quota is easily filled by vegetables, grains and dairy foods. But our main-course meals typically feature much larger amounts—at least 5 or 6 ounces—and we often end up eating them three times a day: bacon or ham with breakfast, tuna salad at lunch and a steak for dinner.

It is thought by many nutritional scientists that high-protein diets work best when augmented with small amounts of carbohydrates. The carbohydrates act to prime the metabolic "pump," assuring that a normal burn-off of fat can occur. When no carbohydrates are available, the body converts to a thrifty starvation metabolism and burns up calories more slowly; this accounts for the weight-loss plateau encountered by those on diets too restricted to protein.

A heavy-protein regimen requires a great deal of water to dilute and wash away the undesirable compounds of protein digestion. That's why people lose weight so quickly at the beginning; in fact, the pounds consist mostly of water, as fluids are drawn out of the body's tissues to meet this ongoing need. Thirst and dehydration can result, along with queasiness—which may also account for some early rapid weight loss: People overdosing on protein may become too sick and nauseous to eat!

PROTEIN PSYCHOLOGY

Animal-protein foods are more expensive than vegetables and are still associated in many minds with prosperity and plenty. Jo Giese Brown, author of *The Good Food Compendium*, illustrates the psychology of protein with the story of some Europeans who after World War II were so delighted to eat meat again (after having been rationed carefully for so long) that they would display a whole ham in their window, whenever they had one, for all their neighbors to see. "A 'ham in the window' became a status symbol, a sign that the family was doing well," the author observes. Eventually everyone wanted a ham, and one person's ingenious idea was to design a lifelike, elegantly painted one out of pottery—for the sole purpose of showing off! The grateful postwar Europeans equated the ham with a return not only to the good life but to superior nutrition as well.

Just like them, many of us have been conditioned to think of the "best" protein as meat, cheese, eggs and milk. All these highly nutritious foods are well represented in Diet Type 2. However, legumes, grains and seeds are also excellent sources; what's more, they're rich in fiber, don't burden you with fats and cholesterol—and are less likely to break down into those not-so-friendly nitrogen waste compounds either. The answer is not to replace one form of protein with another, but to broaden your diet to make room for more healthful choices.

At least half of your daily protein should be from vegetable sources for optimum health, according to the Senate Select Committee on Nutrition. However, almost every diet or nutrition book will claim that animal proteins are "complete," while the vegetable ones are not. Despite evidence to the contrary, this myth persists in the minds of many. The misconception comes largely from an animal study done in the 1920s in which the growth-enhancing foods for rats turned out to be eggs, cheese and milk. The experimenters fed groups of rats different kinds of proteins, one at a time, and then observed how favorably they reacted to each. If a rat responded well, the protein was labeled complete; if not so impressively, it was considered incomplete—period. However, our nutritional needs are markedly different from those of rats. For example, they don't get along very well on human milk, as theirs is about nine times higher in protein than ours. Also, the most up-to-date methods of nutritional analysis have since shown that varied vegetable sources of protein generally contain all the amino acids in sufficient quantities to satisfy human needs. The "complete"/"incomplete" fiction has led to excessively painstaking food combining among people who prefer vegetable proteins but believe they are unable to meet their daily nutritional needs without a lot of elaborate mixing and matching. Even Frances Moore Lappé, the author of the protein-combining orthodoxy, *Diet for a Small Planet,* has since recanted her earlier, more extreme views.

It's hard to believe that an antiquated and misleading rat study could be the primary basis for our *current* protein "policy." Consider this a vivid example of how nutritional misinformation enjoys a charmed shelf life! It's almost impossible to uncover any example of protein deficiency in this country. In anything but the most extreme single-food fad diet, most proteins are combined naturally anyway: Rice and beans, macaroni and cheese, cereal and milk, nut butters and whole-grain bread are common examples. But, I repeat, as long as you're getting enough calories, *it's not necessary to do this consciously.* It's distressing to imagine how many people have shied away from even trying vegetarian cuisine because they feared being shortchanged on protein or thought it took too much trouble to get all the combinations right!

THE MODIFIED PROTEIN ALTERNATIVE

By now you're probably convinced that too much protein is not a good idea and that you should vary the kinds you eat, for the sake of both your appearance and long-term health. But still, your personal profile shows that a protein-based diet works best for you. If you were referred to this section because of your score on the questionnaire, you may simply prefer the taste of protein foods—you swear you'll never be a "vegetable person" or find them more suited to your life-style at home and work. Maybe you've always responded reasonably well to a protein-type plan and wonder how you can make it work even better, without robbing you of energy or essential nutrients or raising your cholesterol unaccept-ably. The answer is to modify and augment the protein diets that are so efficient in the short run at trimming away extra pounds and to turn them to your lifelong advantage. That's where the Modified Protein-Plus Diet, or Diet Type 2, comes in. It contains plenty of protein, but not more than your body needs and *not* at the expense of carbohydrates. Its proteins are also from a variety of sources, including the most benefi-cial animal foods: seafood, free-range poultry and game, low-fat milk and the leanest meats.

Let's look at the truly "superior" proteins, one by one, that will make up this diet and should be the basis for any slimming, life-enhancing plan.

SEAFOOD: THE GREAT CATCH!

In the early 1970s, a team of researchers studying Eskimos in their native Greenland found that though their diets were alarmingly high in fat, they suffered virtually no heart disease, cancer, arthritis, diabetes or any of the other familiar ills of the Western world. How was this possible? It happened that the fats they so freely consumed were almost entirely from whale blubber and raw fish—to the tune of nearly a pound a day. No one is surprised to hear that seafood, rich in protein and low in calories, is highly nutritious and an integral part of a sensible diet. What *is* astonishing is that anything described as "fat" could turn out to be its most healthful, lifesaving component!

Indeed, the Omega-3 fatty acids—a group of polyunsaturates found in seafood—may be nature's underwater miracle drug. Among other benefits, the Omega-3s are known to help decrease serum cholesterol and triglycerides as well as to interfere with the formation of blood clots within arteries, thus altering the process which leads to heart attacks and strokes. Omega-3 fatty acids may also be connected with the prevention of breast cancer and inflammatory diseases such as arthritis. One recent study, which involved 852 men living in the Netherlands, found that as little as two servings of fish per week resulted in a 50 percent reduction in the heart-attack rate.

Regardless of your diet, the cholesterol from the food you eat never travels unescorted. Rather, it circulates through your bloodstream wrapped in a package of protein carriers known as lipoproteins. Low-density and very-low-density lipoproteins (LDLs and VLDLs) are responsible for depositing their cholesterol "cargo" on artery walls, where it can become a permanent fixture, piling up and ultimately blocking the passage of blood. In contrast, high-density lipoproteins, or HDLs, act in a positive way (imagine the H stands for "healthy") as they usher cholesterol away from cells and carry it to the liver for breakdown or removal by the body. People with relatively high HDL levels and thus cleaner arteries are less prone to heart disease. Premenopausal women have more HDLs in their bloodstream than men do, which may explain why they also have fewer premature heart attacks. A diet high in certain polyunsaturates lowers the destructive LDLs, while one dominated by saturated fats does just the opposite.

Until scientists encountered the Omega-3s, almost everyone assumed that vegetable oils were the best sources of these protective, cholesterol-controlling polyunsaturates. As recently as the 1970s, certain nutritional scientists proposed that people drink polyunsaturated vegetable oil as a means of hiking their "P/S ratios" (ratio of dietary polyunsaturated to saturated oils). But the polyunsaturated oils found in seafood may be truly superior. Unfortunately, vegetable polyunsaturates reduce not only the troublemaking LDLs but also the valuable HDLs; they've also been shown to stimulate the growth of tumors in laboratory animals. Seafood oils, however, alter the way the liver synthesizes LDLs and reduce their levels in the body; they also leave the desirable HDLs intact and may even increase them. (The monounsaturates, found in olive and soy oil, are believed to behave in similar fashion.)

Yet another benefit is that, while vegetable oils may increase triglycerides, those in seafood seem to prevent these same artery-clogging substances from being produced in the first place.

Fish oils give all the evidence of preventing another dreaded condition. The Japanese, who obtain half of their fat intake from the sea, have one of the lowest rates of breast cancer in the world. Studies have shown that adding fish oils to the diets of mice reduced the number and size of malignant mammary growths, and scientists speculate that the protection applies to humans as well.

What all this means is that the *fattiest* fish are *best* for you:

Salmon, mackerel, herring, tuna, rainbow trout, halibut, whitefish and sardines are especially rich in Omega-3s. They come from cold, deep-water habitats; the oils act as an anti-freeze in the icy seas, enabling the fish's cells to remain flexible.

Seafood is also a good supplier of the B complex vitamins, important for skin and nervous-system health. In addition, it provides generous amounts of iron, calcium, potassium, trace minerals such as zinc and selenium—both closely related to hormone regulation—and ample protein in easily digestible form.

How much do you need in your diet to reap all the rewards? An average of just ½ pound a week, or two 4-ounce servings, is enough.

When you shop for fresh seafood, make sure it has no tell-tale "fishy" odor; its flesh should be moist, firm and shiny, and the eyes clear and protruding. If you buy frozen fish, take care that it doesn't have ice crystals or freezer burn, and is not partially thawed or contained in damaged packaging. (Fortunately, freezing has no effect on the Omega-3s; cooking and canning have very little.)

Refrigerate fresh seafood in the coldest section as soon as possible and cook it within two days of buying or defrosting for maximum flavor. Store frozen seafood in moisture-proof wrapping, use within two or three months and never refreeze it after it has been thawed. Keep canned seafood in a cool,

ORIENTAL TREATS

Japanese sushi restaurants can provide gourmet eaters with low-cholesterol, high-protein delicacies: raw or steamed fish, such as fresh mackerel and tuna, with low-carbohydrate complements, such as seaweed and a light green salad or sautéed vegetables.

dry place but don't store it longer than a year. If possible buy it water-packed or low in sodium.

For best results with fresh fish, broil quickly at a high temperature: ten minutes for each inch of thickness, at 450 degrees, or until it looks opaque; double the time for frozen fish. Other simple ways to prepare:

- Bake: Place in an oven dish and cover with sauce or a mixture of lemon, olive oil and herbs. Bake at 350 degrees for 15 minutes.
- Poach: Place just enough water, milk or wine to cover in a wide, shallow pan and bring to a boil. Add fish. Cover tightly and simmer about 10 minutes or until done. Add seasoning as desired.
- Steam: In a deep pot, place fish on a steamer rack 2 inches above boiling liquid. Cover tightly, for about 10 minutes or until done.
- Pan fry: Coat with seasoned flour, bread or cracker crumbs and place in ¼ to ½ inch hot olive oil for about 10 minutes or until done.
- Microwave: Allow three minutes per pound for fish fillets, or follow manufacturer's directions.

Fish is ready when it is opaque, not shiny, and doesn't cling to the bone. The American Heart Association urges against using salt for flavoring and suggests relying instead on delicious, fresh alternatives like lemon juice, dill weed, parsley, oregano, basil, rosemary, thyme, marjoram, bay leaf, onion, garlic, tarragon or paprika. As for dry herbs, one-third teaspoon of powder or one-half teaspoon crushed is equivalent to one tablespoon of fresh chopped herbs.

Low-Fat Dairy Foods

Whether or not you're watching your weight, the only dairy products fit to be regularly eaten on the Protein-Plus Diet are low in fat: skim milk, low-fat cottage, pot or farmer cheese, yogurt, goat's milk or cheese (chèvre), the new "lite" versions of many cheeses and low-calorie ice creams. (As for the last, some of the alternatives, including whipped, creamy fruit concoctions and "Rice Dream," are unbelievably delicious and difficult even for diehard connoisseurs to resist!)

Here's a close-up of the best dairy foods and the growing number of choices available to both weight- and health-conscious consumers:

MILK

One 8-ounce glass adds up to 20 percent of your daily protein requirement.

Whole Milk (3.5 percent fat): This is best for infants and small children, and nonoverweight pregnant or breast-feeding women.

Low-Fat or 2-percent Milk: Beware! This is not as low as it sounds. Consider that it more closely resembles whole milk (3.5 percent) than skim, which contains 0 percent fat. It's also closer in calories to the "real thing," with 145 per cup. But it could serve as a halfway step for those who wish to cut back on fat gradually and who find the switch from whole to skim or 1 percent too drastic to make all at once.

Low-Fat or 1-percent Milk (1–1.5 percent fat): This is an improvement, but keep in mind that you still have a better alternative: cutting fat down to near zero. Milk may be good for you, but the whole kind should be an occasional indulgence rather than a daily habit, whether you are trying to lose weight or protect yourself from heart disease.

Skim Milk (.05 percent fat): As long as it's fortified with vitamins A and D, skim milk is more desirable than whole because it provides identical nutritional value without the added fat and calories. It comes with an extra protein boost, too: 1 gram more of protein powder than regular milk per glass to enhance its flavor and texture. You might also try adding a teaspoon or two of instant nonfat dry milk powder to make it thicker and less watery.

Low-Fat Buttermilk: This delicious product is made from low-fat or skim milk and a small amount of added butterfat, nonfat dry milk solids and cultured bacteria. Roughly equivalent to 1 percent milk, it can be used in pancake batter and as a substitute in any recipes calling for whole milk, cream or half-and-half. One cup is about 88 calories.

Lactaid Milk: According to its producer, Lactaid Inc., this is a low-fat milk (1 percent) designed for the lactose-intolerant, in which an added enzyme, lactase, breaks down the lactose into two digestible sugars.

CalciMilk: Low-fat or skim-milk Lactaid fortified with 500 milligrams of calcium per cup.

Ultrapastureurized Milk: Some cream and milk is now being ultrapasteurized, or heated for about two seconds at very high temperatures (above 290°F), which not only kills disease-producing bacteria but most of the ones responsible for spoilage, too. Thus treated, milk and cream can be refrigerated for as long as two months, compared to the usual ten or twelve days. Though convenient, ultrapasteurization may rob milk of certain heat-labile nutrients.

Acidophilus Cultured Milk: Pasteurized or ultrapasteurized (usually low-fat or skim) milk combined with a concentrated culture of lactobacillus acidophilus. Research has shown that this bacterium aids the digestive process.

Dry Nonfat Milk: Pasteurized skim milk with all the water removed. It's made by spraying hot dry air into concentrated skim milk. Vitamins A and D are added. It can be combined with meat loaf and ground meats for extra calcium without altering the taste. It has a convenient shelf life of one year.

Yogurt: When whole, skim or part-skim milk is fermented with a special bacterial culture, the result is yogurt. It has the same nutritional value as its milk base, but it's easier to digest and poses no problem for the lactose-intolerant. The plain, low-fat kind (to which you may add fresh fruit) is best; fruit flavors contain added sugar. Dannon, Colombo, Weight Watchers and other manufacturers have recently introduced *nonfat* plain and flavored yogurts, virtually devoid of fat and cholesterol, yet smooth and piquant. Caution: Store-bought frozen yogurt is no calorie bargain. The vanilla version, for example, has more sugar than vanilla ice cream and about the same number of calories (250 per 8-ounce serving). But it does contain less fat: 2 percent, as compared to 10 percent.

Kefir: This fermented milk product is low in fat (1.5 percent), tangy, rich in protein and B vitamins and even higher in calcium than yogurt. It's also lower in sugar and calories and just as easy to digest since it contains microorganisms that break milk sugar (lactose) into lactic acid.

Low-Fat Cheeses: America's favorite food comes in a wide variety of healthful forms today. There are part-skim and low-fat cheeses, reduced-calorie and low-sodium cheddar, mozzarella, cream, ricotta and cottage cheese, among many others. Most of the selections are excellent and the taste differences are imperceptible even to the fussiest palates.

Cheese is naturally nourishing, high in calcium, protein, riboflavin, vitamin A and zinc. Unfortunately, about 65 to 75 percent of its calories come from saturated fat. A typical 1½-ounce serving contains about as much fat as 3½ pats of butter! While part-skim sounds like a responsible choice, it's often not much leaner than its whole-milk counterpart. For example, part-skim mozzarella contains only 25 percent less fat than the regular kind (still totaling a whopping 51 percent), and part-skim ricotta has 10 grams of fat per half cup—hardly a low-fat alternative by any standard. The only varieties that are naturally low in fat are pot, farmer, goat and dry-curd or 1-percent cottage cheese.

Without adequate fat, most cheeses become dry and rock-hard; sapsago, which some people find unpalatable, is a common example. To overcome the problem, manufacturers can use water to replace the moisture-giving fat, resulting in a processed (not technically "natural") cheese. The catch is that some of these are exceedingly high in sodium (typically 450 to 700 milligrams per serving), since this is added to keep the ingredients from separating during processing. One notable exception is Weight Watchers Reduced Sodium (Low-Fat) Cheese Product, with only 140 milligrams of sodium and 2 grams of fat per serving.

"Sapsago, cottage [type] and processed products aside, it's pointless to search for a truly low-fat cheese," observes Bonnie Liebman in a recent issue of *The Nutrition Action Newsletter.** "Your best bet is to compensate by slashing fat elsewhere in your diet, or by keeping servings small," she adds. "In sandwiches, use one slice rather than two or three. For casseroles, try adding grated cheese only where it shows. With luck, only your arteries will notice that the inside isn't oozing with fat."

The following chart lists popular low-fat cheeses according to their fat, calcium and sodium content.

―――――――――――――――――■―――――――――――――――――

LOW-FAT CHEESES†

Variety	Serving Size (ounces)	Calories	Fat (grams)	Calcium (milli- grams)	Serving Suggestions
American Flavor *Pasteurized Process*					Use for sandwiches.
Light n' Lively (Kraft)	1	70	4	199	
Lite-line (Borden)	1	50	2	200	
Weight Watchers	1	50	2	150	

* February 1986, published by the Center for Science in the Public Interest, Washington, D.C.

† Reprinted by permission of the National Dairy Council and based on information from the U.S. Dept. of Agriculture.

Variety	Serving Size (ounces)	Calories	Fat (grams)	Calcium (milligrams)	Serving Suggestions
Bonbel *Reduced Calorie*	1	60	4	209	Mild flavor, similar to Edam. Use for snacks, dessert, with fruit.
Cheddar *Natural Cheddar Style*					Mild to sharp flavor. Use for snacks, sandwiches, casseroles, sauces, on pie.
Heidi Ann	1	83	5	200	
Ryser	1	83	5	200	
Tendale	1	70	4	260	
Weight Watchers	1	80	5	200	
Pasteurized Process					
Light n' Lively (Kraft) Sharp Cheddar Flavor	1	72	5	192	
Lite-line (Borden) Mild Cheddar Flavor	1	50	2	200	
Sharp Cheddar Flavor	1	50	2	200	
Cheese Food *Sharp Cheddar*					Use for snacks, sandwiches, casseroles, with fruit, for dessert.
May-bud	1	70	4	150	
Weight Watchers	1	70	4	200	
Colby Flavor *Pasteurized Process*					Mild to mellow flavor. Use for salads, sandwiches, snacks.
Lite-line (Borden)	1	50	2	200	

Variety	Serving Size (ounces)	Calories	Fat (grams)	Calcium (milli- grams)	Serving Suggestions
Cottage Cheese					Mild table cheese. Use for salads, dips, baking.
Creamed	4	117	5	68	
Low Fat, 2% Fat	4	101	2	77	
Cream Cheese					Use for sandwich spreads, dips, salads, with bagels.
Light Philadelphia Brand	1	60	5	31	
Weight Watchers (Reduced Calorie)	1	30	1	20	
Farmer Cheese *Natural*					Clean, mild flavor. Use for salads, snacks, cooking.
May-bud	1	90	2	150	
Simon's	1	80	5	200	
Monterey Jack Flavor *Pasteurized Process*					Mild to mellow flavor. Use for salads, sandwiches, Mexican cooking.
Lite-line (Borden)	1	50	2	200	
Mozzarella					Mild flavor. Use for pizza, lasagna, grilled sandwiches.
Natural (Part Skim)	1	72	5	183	
Pasteurized Process					
Lite-line (Borden)	1	50	2	200	
Muenster Flavor *Pasteurized Process*					A semisoft cheese with a mild to mellow flavor. Use for snacks, sandwiches.
Lite-line (Borden)	1	50	2	200	

Variety	Serving Size (ounces)	Calories	Fat (grams)	Calcium (milli- grams)	Serving Suggestions
Ricotta					Semisweet flavor. Use for cooked dishes, salads, dips, fillings, desserts.
Natural (Part Skim)	1	43	3	84	
Natural (Whole Milk)	1	54	4	65	
Scamorze *Natural (Part Skim)*					Mild flavor. Use for cooking Italian dishes.
Jewel	1	79	5	200	
Falbo	1	80	5	200	
String Cheese *Natural*					Mild flavor. Use for snacks.
Kraft (Part Skim)	1	82	5	212	
Falbo	1	80	5	200	
Tolibia	1	80	5	200	
Swiss Flavor *Pasteurized Process*					Mild, nutty, sweet flavor. Use for sandwiches, salads, fondues, casseroles.
Light n' Lively (Kraft)	1	71	4	214	
Lite-line (Borden)	1	50	2	200	

EGGS

Unless you and your family have a history of high cholesterol and/or heart disease, it's okay to eat two or three eggs a week. According to a recent study at the Radcliffe Infirmary in Oxford, England, when subjects on a normal diet were given extra eggs, they showed no significant changes in their blood cholesterol.

Most important, they concurrently ate more fiber and reduced their intake of saturated fats. Apparently, for most people on otherwise healthful diets, the body excretes the cholesterol it cannot use, or else cuts down on the amount it produces on its own. However, since saturated fat is often converted into cholesterol by the body, curbing its amount can make a marked difference. Sure enough, the British study showed that a substantial drop in blood cholesterol occurred when the participants initially switched to the low-fat diet.

While a few whole eggs a week won't thicken your waistline or shorten your life, remember the "invisible" yolks found in cakes, egg noodles, mayonnaise, some yogurts, frozen waffles and other prepared foods, or the ones called for in your favorite recipes. If you are doing the cooking or baking, substitute one and a half or two egg whites for each whole egg required. Commercial egg substitutes contain dangerous levels of hydrogenated fats, which themselves pose risks to your heart.

MEAT

Condemned for its heart-threatening fats and cholesterol, its cancer-promoting additives, red meat has taken a beating in recent years. But it is now reappearing in slimmed-down form, its image remarkably improved. Our national craving for healthier food has spurred some farmers to fatten their cattle with natural foods like pesticide-free alfalfa, corn and grass, and to crossbreed them with leaner livestock. The results are some custom meats with up to 85 percent less fat and 80 percent fewer calories than standard beef. Of course, for those with a tendency to high cholesterol, red meat remains a questionable choice.

The newest data from the U.S. Department of Agriculture put beef in the same nutritional ballpark as chicken: A well-trimmed 3-ounce sirloin has 185 calories and 75 milligrams of cholesterol; a 3-ounce piece of boneless chicken breast totals 140 calories and 72 milligrams of cholesterol. In addition, "natural" beef, which comes from cattle not fed antibiotics, growth hormones, steroids or chemical-free additives, is showing up alongside the leaner alternative.

While the new "light" and "natural" trends are encouraging, the terms can sometimes be misleading. For example, processors who reduce the fat content of their meat by 25 percent can qualify for a "light" label even if the product is still high in fat. "Natural" may mean that nothing was added after the animal was slaughtered; it doesn't guarantee anything about the way it was raised or fed.

Right now, the Nutritional Effects Foundation, a nationwide group founded by cattlemen in 1986, is trying to establish for beef a label similar to the Good Housekeeping Seal of Approval. An NEF stamp would tell doctors and consumers that the meat conforms to American Heart Association guidelines for healthy diets. Many supermarkets now display charts that list the calorie, sodium, fat, cholesterol, vitamin and protein content of their meats alongside dietary standards recommended by the American Heart Association. This new meat "NutriFacts" program also highlights meats with fewer than 200 calories per 3-ounce cooked serving. Some of these include pork tenderloin, with 141 calories; beef top round, with 166; and lamb loin chop, with 188.

Ironically, the more money you pay for meat, the fattier it is. "Prime" meats, the gourmet's delight, are juicy, tender and great-looking precisely because of their extra fat content. "Choice" or "good" cuts of beef are leaner and cheaper. Well-aged eye round tastes as good as rib roasts and T-bones, but has much less fat, fewer calories and no bone. For hamburger, ground sirloin and round have the lowest amounts of fat (10 and 15 percent respectively), but your best bet is to select lean cuts of meat, trim the fat carefully, put the meat in a meat grinder or food processor and add spices to taste. The chart below lists the lowest-fat cuts of meat.

CHART*

MEAT:	(ask for "good" rather than "choice," "choice" rather than "prime") Lowest-fat cuts:
Beef:	Top round steak Round roast Wedge-bone sirloin steak Top loin steak, tenderloin steak, eye round, tip round; brisket, point portion; bottom round steak, chuck arm pot roast
Veal:	Cutlet, arm steak
Pork:	Centerloin chop, shank portion, leg, rump portion, whole leg, shoulder, arm picnic
Lamb:	Shank portion, leg, sirloin portion, foreshank

* Information provided by the National Livestock and Meat Board, Chicago, Illinois.

A BIG BEEF

Frankfurters, which can be up to 30 percent fat or 90 percent water and 5 percent corn syrup and fillers, have little redeeming nutritional value. The "100 percent beef" label on the package does not mean the franks contain no fat or other meat byproducts such as hooves, snouts or entrails—only that there is no other kind of meat in them. Other processed meats, even higher in fat, are less desirable still. A quarter-pound of bologna or salami has 300 calories.

If you must, try chicken or turkey franks, which are lower in fat. Nitrate-free varieties are available at health-food stores and some butcher and gourmet shops.

POULTRY

Chicken producers like Perdue and Holly Farms are turning out skinnier birds these days, although the actual amount of fat you are spared is very little—about a half teaspoon per serving. Most poultry fat is found in the skin and stomach, parts you can easily trim away yourself. Fortunately, birds contain a high proportion of monounsaturated fat (the same kind found in olive oil), which may lower blood cholesterol. Poultry is also relatively low in saturated fat.

Removing the skin makes a decided difference. For example, a 3½-ounce serving of unskinned chicken is 216 calories, with 4.5 grams of saturated fat; without the skin, however, that same portion is only 111 calories, with .4 grams of saturated fat. Even a Peking duck's portly 39 grams of fat per 3½-ounce serving drops down to only 6 grams when the skin is removed. Poultry's light meat alone contains about 22 grams of protein. The dark meat is slightly fattier, but it also has about a quarter more iron. Both provide plenty of B vitamins and a fair share of zinc, copper, manganese and other important trace elements.*

Poultry is also becoming safer to eat, producers claim, as they are learning to rely less on human antibiotics such as penicillin and streptomycin and more on better nutrition and breeding methods to stimulate growth. People who regularly eat medicated animals may become less responsive to the same antibiotics when these are needed to fight an infection. Frequently ingesting antibiotics may also create an imbalance in our bodies' internal bacteria, making us more receptive to salmonella and related diseases. Yet another risk is that animals treated intensively with antibiotics may develop highly drug-resistant strains of bacteria that can infect eaters and are harder to combat with available medications.

Some people believe it's worth paying more for free-range

* See *American Health* magazine, November 1986, pp. 99-110.

poultry: birds that are allowed to graze outdoors on natural wild grasses, herbs and feed and are less frequently treated with antibiotics. They are superior tasting and typically have a higher proportion of unsaturated to saturated fat.

Farm-raised and wild game, including quail, pheasant, squab, rabbit and venison, is increasingly popular, too. Even hard-to-track-down buffalo, wood pigeon, partridge and grouse can be found in specialty butcher shops and on restaurant menus across the U.S. In general, moist, young meat (quail, squab, tender cuts of venison) can be simply roasted or grilled, as you would chicken and steak. When the flesh is older or less tender, stewing or braising are better methods.

Furred or feathered, wild game is enjoying a major revival not only for its taste and native heritage, but also because it

THE SCOOP ON SALMONELLA

Thirty to fifty percent of all chickens and seventy-five percent of all turkeys have salmonella. Fortunately, the bacterium is killed quite easily at natural roasting temperatures. But preparing a raw bird on a cutting board or counter and then failing to thoroughly wash the surface, the utensils or your hands can allow the remaining salmonella organisms to infect another food. Tasting while preparing is highly unsafe. Simply cleaning up after your fowl is in the oven can prevent the disease. Beware, too, the incomplete sterilization that microwave cooking affords. Since heating is from the inside out, microwave heat sensors can show meat is cooked before all parts have reached safe temperatures. A recent study revealed live salmonella organisms in nearly one half of microwaved chickens!

A PROTEIN PLUS

Good news for animal-protein lovers: Lean fish, poultry and meat contain *heme* iron, the type that is most readily absorbed and used by the body.

---

is highly nutritious. Compared to well-marbled beef, with up to 45 percent fat, it usually has no more than 5–7 percent. Even better, much of that fat is in the form of heart-favoring Omega-3 polyunsaturates. This is probably the reason so little atherosclerosis and degenerative disease has been found in today's primitive tribes that rely heavily on game. Indeed, a recent study of the diet of prehistoric man published in the prestigious *New England Journal of Medicine* noted that ancient hunters' diets were rich in Omega-3 fatty acids provided by the grass-fed land animals they ate.

THE SOY-FOODS REVOLUTION: TOFU AND MORE

If you have been to a health-food store lately, you must have noticed all the soy-based goodies lining freezer and shelf: tofu burgers, tofu "pups," "soysage," "soy milk," "tofuna" salad, tempeh Reuben sandwiches, tempeh burgers and chips, tofu cheesecake, pizza and lasagna—almost every favorite food imaginable in a meatless version. All these ingenious creations derive from the same raw material: the soybean, an incredibly versatile, high-protein plant.

Soybean curd, or tofu, is the result of mashing soybeans into soy milk and pressing the mixture into a solid, square-shaped cake. Custardlike to firm in texture, it takes on the flavor of the food it's teamed with. One two-inch square has the same amount of protein as an 8-ounce glass of milk, without the saturated fat and cholesterol. Tofu also has one of the lowest ratios of calories to protein found in any known plant food (about 12 calories per gram of protein). A 4-ounce serving supplies up to 25 percent of the adult RDA for protein, 20 percent of the iron and 20 percent of the phosphorus.

Made from tender cooked beans, tempeh is a fermented soybean patty with a nutty aroma and a soft, chewy, almost meatlike texture. Fresh tempeh has even more protein than tofu, or about as much as beef and chicken.

Miso, made from soybeans, salt, water and often rice or barley, is a fermented seasoning or condiment, somewhat salty, with a pasty consistency similar to that of peanut butter. It's used as a broth base and as a topping for grains and vegetables.

Like other plant proteins, soy foods can be an acquired taste: Try varying your meals with these meat alternatives to enjoy their naturally low-fat, cholesterol-reducing benefits.

LEGUMES: BEANS AND PEAS

The plant kingdom's richest sources of protein are totally free of saturated fat. Their only drawback is that they contain trypsin inhibitors, which interfere with the effects of digestive enzymes. See page 79 for tips on how to make such foods more digestible. Lentils and lima, kidney, alfalfa and mung beans can all be sprouted.

LEGUMES: FOUR EASY STEPS

1. Rinse, and pick out stems or stones.
2. Put legumes in a large pot. Add enough water to cover them.

(Continued)

(*Continued*)

3. Cover the pot and put it in the refrigerator to soak overnight. Or, to save time, boil the legumes for two minutes, then soak for one hour.
4 Cook legumes using directions on package label. (1 cup dry legumes = 2½ cups cooked)

Note: Lentils and split peas do not need to be soaked before cooking.

HIGH-CARBOHYDRATE VEGETABLES

Some vegetables are especially high in carbohydrates and calories. While you're on the Protein-Plus Diet, you might want to eat the following items in moderation only:

- chili peppers, green or red
- sweet potatoes and potatoes
- Chinese water chestnuts
- butternut and acorn squash
- turnip greens
- dandelion greens
- Jerusalem artichokes
- kidney beans, red or white
- parsley
- green onions
- Chinese pea pods
- split peas
- corn on the cob

REMINDER: ELIMINATE EXCESS FAT!

Saturated fats contribute most to cholesterol formation; polyunsaturated fats, the least. However, there is no evidence that the latter help prevent heart disease; on the other hand, once inside the body, they may generate possibly carcinogenic particles known as free radicals. (Laboratory studies have shown an elevated incidence of cancer in subjects fed unsaturated fats.) While vitamin E can inhibit the damage, most of it is lost when oils are processed or refined, so other food sources of the vitamin, such as whole grains and leafy greens, and/or supplements are advised. The best advice, however, is to cut back on all fats as much as possible to reduce your risks of both heart disease and cancer.

WHAT ABOUT FIBER?

On the Modified Protein-Plus Diet your chief sources of fiber will be fruits, vegetables and legumes, plus 1–2 tablespoons of oat or wheat bran, psyllium seeds or a fiber supplement like Metamucil or guar gum with a full glass of water about a half hour before meals. Inadequate fiber has been associated with such diseases as diverticulitis and cancer of the colon. Also, the more bulk in your diet, the less likely you are to overeat.

———————— ▪ ————————

SAMPLE MENUS

Recipes are provided for all dishes marked with an asterisk (*). To find recipes that appear in other sections, consult the Index at the back of this book.

Beverages for all meals: herbal tea, black coffee, instant grain coffee (e.g., Caffix), skim milk, soy milk, seltzer, plain or sparkling mineral water, fresh vegetable juices or filtered tap water.

DAY 1:

Breakfast

1 soft-boiled or sunny-side-up egg on toasted whole-wheat English muffin

½ grapefruit

Lunch

1 serving Spicy Tuna-Vegetable Melt*

1 cup skim milk

1 apple

Dinner

4 ounces broiled loin lamb chop with mint *or* Magic Meat Loaf*

Stir-fry vegetables with Tahini-Miso Dressing*

Mixed green salad with tarragon vinegar and 1 teaspoon olive oil

Snacks

1 tablespoon roasted pumpkin seeds

½ cup low-fat (1 percent) cottage cheese with chopped scallions, radishes and green peppers with dash of hot sauce

DAY 2:

Breakfast

High-Protein Shake*

Lunch

Turkey Salad with Raw Vegetable Platter*

Dinner

4 ounces Broiled (or Poached) Salmon with Dill and Lemon Sauce*

½ cup each steamed carrots and turnip greens

Chilled mandarin orange slices with ½ cup plain low-fat yogurt

Snack

8-ounce glass kefir (low-fat cultured milk)

DAY 3:

Breakfast

Farmer Cheese with Cinnamon and Apples* on toast

Lunch

½ cup Great Chickpea Spread*

Cucumber, onion and tomato salad

Dinner

4 ounces Skinless Breast of Chicken*

String beans sautéed with garlic and 1 tablespoon olive oil

½ cup steamed broccoli, cabbage and cauliflower with fresh herbs and 1 teaspoon sesame seeds

Snacks

2 rice cakes with 1 teaspoon Enhanced Butter Herb Spread*

DAY 4:

Breakfast

Scrambled Tofu with Turmeric and Scallions* *or* 1 soft-boiled egg with 1 slice rye toast

Lunch

4 ounces broiled chicken (with sautéed vegetables, if desired) *or* 4 ounces canned water-packed seafood

Baked potato with low-fat cottage cheese, chives and parsley

Dinner

4–6 ounces Broiled Bluefish*

Mixed green salad with mandarin orange slices

Snack

1 ounce goat cheese on Ry-Krisp or Wasa cracker

DAY 5:

Breakfast

1 cup plain low-fat yogurt or vanilla kefir with assorted fresh fruit

Lunch

4 ounces Deep-Sea Fish Cakes* *or* Finnish Pickled Herring*

Escarole and chicory salad with Velvety Tofu Dressing*

Dinner

4 ounces Enchanted Stuffed Cornish Game Hen*

½ cup Broccoli Italian Style (sautéed with 2 teaspoons olive oil, fresh minced garlic, hot red pepper flakes; cooked, covered, for 10 minutes; served with lemon juice or wine vinegar)

Snack

1 tablespoon roasted (unsalted) sunflower seeds

DAY 6:

Breakfast

Light Western Omelet*

1 thin slice seven-grain bread

8 ounces fresh-squeezed citrus or unsalted tomato juice

Lunch

4 ounces pasta with seafood, vegetables or meatless tomato sauce

½ cup fresh strawberries or other fruit in season with low-fat plain yogurt

Dinner

4 ounces Fancy Baked Mackerel* *or* Very Lean Pepper Steak with Onions*

½ cup steamed spinach with garlic, olive oil, herbs and sesame seeds

Snack

1 ounce low-fat cheese on Kavli crackers

DAY 7:

Breakfast

Low-Cal Welsh Rarebit*

Lunch

4 ounces light-meat poultry (preferably without skin) *or* Filet of Sole Almondine*

Cucumber salad with chopped scallions, 1 tablespoon each olive oil and white vinegar

Dinner

4 ounces Curry Chicken (or Shrimp) with Vegetables and Rice*

Steamed asparagus spears with lemon juice and ½ pat melted butter

Snacks

2 rice cakes with 2 teaspoons natural unsalted peanut butter

———————▪———————

FIVE EASY PIECES

Satisfying, nutritious, portable lunch/dinner alternatives that you can prepare with a minimum of fuss and effort. Each makes one individual portion.

1. *Curry salmon*
   Fork-blend one 3½-ounce individual can water-packed salmon, white of 1 hard-boiled egg, 1 tablespoon finely chopped dill pickle and pinch of curry to taste. Slice tomato in half, scoop out and stuff with salmon mix.

2. *Oriental poultry salad*
   Dice 3 ounces cooked white turkey meat or skinless breast of chicken. Add ¼ cucumber sliced matchstick style, ½ teaspoon low-sodium soy sauce, ½ teaspoon dark sesame oil, juice of ¼ lemon and pinch of ginger powder or chopped fresh ginger. Serve on a bed of romaine lettuce.

3. *Quick stuffed peppers*
   Mix ¼ cup chickpeas, 1 tablespoon natural peanut butter and pinch of garlic powder; mash thoroughly with fork. Slice 1 large red pepper into quarters, discard seeds and stuff quarters with mixture.

4. *Hold-the-mayo tuna salad*
   Fork-blend one 3½-ounce individual can water-packed tuna with 2 tablespoons low-fat plain yogurt and ½ finely grated carrot. Serve on bed of lettuce or on rice crackers; garnish with alfalfa sprouts.

5. *Egg salad nouveau*
   Fork-blend whites and one yolk of two hard-boiled eggs with 2 tablespoons low-fat plain yogurt and ½ chopped scallion. Serve in celery or on Kavli Norwegian flatbread.

———————▪———————

———————————— ▪ ————————————

RECIPES

Spicy tuna-vegetable melt   *1st Day Lunch*

4 ounces canned, water-packed tuna fish
½ cup sautéed chopped onions
½ cup finely chopped parboiled string beans and carrots
1 slice low-fat cheese
1 fresh tomato, sliced

Preheat oven to 350 degrees. In small casserole dish, mix tuna with sautéed chopped onion and parboiled vegetables. Top with cheese slice and sliced tomato. Bake 4–6 minutes, until cheese is melted. *Serves 2.*

Magic meat loaf   *1st Day Dinner*

½ cup defatted beef or chicken broth
1 cup whole-wheat bread crumbs
¾ pound lean ground beef
¼ pound texturized vegetable protein (TVP)
1 onion, finely chopped
1 clove garlic, pressed
1 tablespoon grated horseradish
½ grated carrot
3 egg whites
¼ teaspoon oregano
¼ teaspoon basil

Preheat oven to 350 degrees. Cook broth in saucepan and bring to a boil. Slowly add bread crumbs and stir till crumbs absorb the broth. Put beef and TVP into a bowl with breadcrumb mixture. Add onion, pressed garlic, horseradish, carrot, eggs and seasonings. Mix with a wooden spoon until well blended.

Grease ovenproof loaf pan and press in the meat loaf mixture. Bake for 45 minutes. *Serves 4.*

Tahini-miso dressing   *1st Day Dinner*

½ cup tahini
2 cloves garlic
1 cup water
¼ cup lemon juice
2 tablespoons miso
2 tablespoons tamari (soy) sauce

Blend ingredients together in a blender. Add more water if mixture is too thick. *Yield: approximately 2 cups.*

High-protein shake   *2nd Day Breakfast*

½ cup plain low- or nonfat yogurt
1 cup skim milk
¼ teaspoon vanilla
1 tablespoon lecithin granules
1 teaspoon wheat germ oil
½ ripe banana
Pinch of cinnamon
1 tablespoon carob powder
1 tablespoon protein powder
1 teaspoon brewer's yeast

Place all ingredients into blender. Blend until totally mixed and frothy. Serve cold. *Serves 2.*

Turkey salad with raw vegetable platter   2nd Day Lunch

4 ounces cooked white turkey meat, diced
1 tablespoon Weight Watchers mayonnaise
1 celery stalk, finely diced
¼ red onion, diced
⅛ teaspoon curry
Pinch of sage
Salt and pepper to taste

Mix all ingredients together. Serve on a bed of lettuce.
Serves 2.

Suggested Raw Vegetables:
Carrot slices
Radishes
Green and red pepper slices
Cucumber or zucchini slices
Raw broccoli or cauliflower

Broiled salmon with dill and lemon sauce   2nd Day Dinner

4–6 ounces fresh salmon
Juice of 1 lemon
1½ tablespoons olive oil
1 clove garlic, minced
1 teaspoon dill
Pinch of salt

Baste salmon with mixture of lemon, olive oil and seasonings. Place in broiler on medium heat (350 degrees). Cook until tender. *Serves 1.*

Farmer cheese with cinnamon and apples   3rd Day Breakfast

4 ounces low-fat farmer cheese
½ cooked apple

Pinch of cinnamon
1 slice toasted whole-wheat bread

Mix cheese, apple and cinnamon and place on toast. Place in broiler for 1–2 minutes. Watch closely. Serve hot with knife and fork. *Serves 1.*

Great chickpea spread   3rd Day Lunch

1 cup cooked or canned chickpeas
¼ cup cooking or canning liquid from beans
½ cup plain low-fat yogurt
½ cup grated or finely chopped onion
½ clove garlic, minced
1 tablespoon lemon juice
¼ teaspoon cumin
1 tablespoon chopped fresh parsley

Combine everything in a blender. Add more liquid if necessary. Spread on thin crackers (Kavli flatbread). Top with mixed sprouts. *Serves 4.*

Skinless breast of chicken   3rd Day Dinner

2 tablespoons olive oil
2 teaspoons lemon juice
½ teaspoon oregano
1 clove garlic, finely chopped
4 ounces organic or free-range chicken breast
½ cup wheat germ or oat bran

Preheat oven to 350 degrees. Combine oil, lemon juice, oregano and garlic. Pound chicken into cutlet and dip into seasoning mixture. Coat chicken pieces with wheat germ or oat bran by shaking together in paper bag. Bake in oiled casserole dish for 25 minutes. *Serves 1.*

Enhanced butter herb spread   *3rd Day Snack*

½ cup lightly salted butter
½ cup olive oil (cold-pressed)
2 pinches of parsley
Pinch of cardamom
Pinch of dill
2 teaspoons lecithin granules
1 tablespoon water

Place all ingredients in blender and blend on high for approximately 1 minute. Spread on crackers, bread, rice cakes, etc. *Yield: 1 cup*

Scrambled tofu with turmeric and scallions   *4th Day Breakfast*

2 teaspoons olive oil
12 ounces tofu, crumbled
½ scallion, finely diced
1 teaspoon tamari (soy) sauce
⅓ teaspoon turmeric
¼ teaspoon basil

Heat pan on medium flame; lightly coat with oil. Add tofu, scallion and tamari; stir. Let cook for 2–3 minutes. Add herbs, stirring frequently for 2–3 minutes more. *Serves 2–3.*

Broiled bluefish   *4th Day Dinner*

4 ounces bluefish
2 tomato slices
Pinch of paprika
Salt and pepper to taste

Top fish with tomato slices. Season to taste. Broil until fish is flaky (about 10 minutes). Garnish with lemon wedges. *Serves 1.*

Deep-sea fish cakes   *5th Day Lunch*

1 pound boiled, peeled
   potatoes
2 tablespoons Enhanced
   Butter Herb Spread (see
   page 160)
2 tablespoons buttermilk
7½ ounces water-packed
   sardines, salmon or tuna
2 lemons
¼ teaspoon paprika
¼ teaspoon marjoram
½ teaspoon sage
4 egg whites
2 tablespoons oat flour
½ cup dried whole-wheat
   bread crumbs
Olive oil
Parsley
Lettuce

Mash potatoes with butter and buttermilk. Drain seafood, mash and add to potatoes. Add the juice of one lemon, and add seasonings. Mix in 2 egg whites.

Preheat oven to 350 degrees. Put remaining 2 egg whites in a separate bowl. Put oat flour and bread crumbs on separate plates. Make 8 flat patties from fish mixture. Dip first in flour, then in egg white, then coat lightly with bread crumbs. Lightly oil baking pan. Add patties and bake about 20 minutes until they are lightly browned on both sides. Garnish with parsley, lettuce and lemon wedges. *Serves 4.*

Finnish pickled herring   *5th Day Lunch*

---

4 fresh herring fillets
3 onions, sliced
½ cup hot water
1¼ cup apple cider vinegar
¼ cup apple juice
2 bay leaves
¼ teaspoon mustard seed powder
⅛ teaspoon cloves
¼ teaspoon allspice
3 whole peppercorns

Wash herring thoroughly. Put in a bowl with cold water, and cover and soak 24 hours, changing water more than twice. Drain, cut off heads and cut each fish into 4 pieces. Place with onions in a large jar or container that can be covered. Combine hot water, cider vinegar, apple juice and spices. Stir well. Pour over the herring. Cover and marinate in the refrigerator for at least 24 hours. Remove bay leaves. Serve cold. *Serves 6.*

Velvety tofu dressing   *5th Day Lunch*

---

6 ounces tofu
2 tablespoons lemon juice
2 tablespoons linseed oil or walnut oil
½ teaspoon curry powder
2 tablespoons minced onion

Combine in a blender and puree. Keep refrigerated. Will keep for 3 days. *Yield: 1 cup.*

Enchanted stuffed Cornish game hens   *5th Day Dinner*

2 Cornish game hens
¼ teaspoon rosemary
¼ teaspoon thyme
1 tablespoon Enhanced
   Butter Herb Spread (see
   page 160)
½ cup chopped onion
2 cups chopped bok choy
¼ cup vegetable broth
2 tablespoons white
   cooking wine
4 slices whole-wheat bread,
   cut into small cubes
½ teaspoon sage
Fresh ground pepper to
   taste

Preheat oven to 400 degrees. Remove all fat from inside of hens. Sprinkle rosemary and thyme on hens.

Stuffing:
Melt Enhanced Butter in skillet. Add onion and bok choy. Sauté and stir 1–2 minutes, coating vegetables with butter. Add broth, cooking another 3 minutes. Add wine and cook 1 minute more. Remove from heat. Stir in bread cubes, sage and pepper to taste.

Place ¼ of the stuffing into each bird's cavity. Close the cavity with string or skewers, tying legs together. Place remaining stuffing in an ovenproof pan and set aside. Fold the wings back and place the birds, legs up, in a shallow baking pan greased with olive oil. Roast hens for 50 minutes; place extra stuffing in oven 25 minutes into cooking time. Cut hens in half lengthwise and serve. Skin may be removed after cooking to reduce fat. *Serves 4.*

Light western omelet   **6th Day Breakfast**

1 egg
2 egg whites
Dash of skim or low-fat milk
⅓ green pepper, chopped
½ small onion, chopped
1 teaspoon olive oil
Pinch of salt
Pinch of cayenne pepper
1 tablespoon finely diced precooked ham slice (optional)

Beat eggs and milk with fork. Sauté vegetables in oil with salt, pepper and ham (if desired) until golden; set aside. Place egg mixture in omelet or frying pan over medium heat. As soon as eggs begin to congeal, place vegetable filling on top and to one side of eggs; gently flip other half of eggs over to cover filling. Lower heat. Cover pan and cook until desired consistency is reached. Serve hot. *Serves 2.*

Fancy baked mackerel   **6th Day Dinner**

2 mackerel filets, unskinned
1 onion, thinly sliced
1½ cups chopped fresh tomatoes, (drain extra liquid)
¼ teaspoon ground coriander
¼ teaspoon fresh chopped or dried basil
¼ teaspoon oregano
¼ teaspoon ground fennel (optional)
1 small clove garlic, finely chopped
¾ tablespoon olive oil

Preheat oven to 350 degrees. Wash mackerel. Layer pieces in baking dish. Place onion slices on top of fish. Combine all other ingredients; pour over fish. Bake uncovered for 45 minutes to 1 hour until fish is tender. *Serves 3.*

Very lean pepper steak with onions　　　*6th Day Dinner*

1 pound very lean steak
1 medium onion, finely chopped
2 tablespoons olive oil
Thinly sliced green and red peppers, shredded cabbage,
　　finely chopped broccoli, cauliflower and/or any other raw
　　vegetables
½ teaspoon each, thyme, marjoram

Remove all visible fat from steak and broil to desired doneness. Sauté onion in oil until it turns transparent; add water to pan if oil dries up. Toss in assorted chopped vegetables and spices and sauté for several minutes. Top steak with mixture and fresh ground pepper. *Serves 4.*

Low-cal welsh rarebit　　　*7th Day Breakfast*

4 slices whole-wheat bread
Small amount Enhanced Butter Herb Spread (see page 160)
¼ pound low-fat or part-skim hard cheese
¼ teaspoon ground mace
Pinch of powdered mustard
2 tablespoons "lite" beer
Pinch of pepper

Preheat oven to 375 degrees. Toast bread and butter the slices *sparingly* with Enhanced Butter Herb Spread while hot. Cut cheese into cubes. Place bread on baking sheets. Put cheese in a saucepan with mace, mustard and beer. Cook over low heat, stirring with wooden spoon until cheese melts and is creamy. Spread mixture over toast. Sprinkle with pepper and bake 10 minutes. *Serves 2.*

Filet of sole almondine   *7th Day Lunch*

6 ounces fresh filet of sole
Sliced almonds
Freshly chopped dill
Lemon wedges
Fresh ground pepper

Arrange fish and almonds with chopped dill on top in broiling pan. Broil until fish becomes flaky (approximately 3–4 minutes, but keep an eye on it). Squeeze lemon over fish while still hot. Pepper to taste. *Serves 2.*

Curry chicken with vegetables and rice   *7th Day Dinner*

1 pound chicken, skinned and cut into pieces
½ teaspoon ginger
½ teaspoon basil
Pinch of paprika
1½ teaspoons Enhanced
    Butter Herb Spread (see page 160)
1 onion, chopped
¼ cup chopped scallion
¼ cup chopped celery
1 cup chopped broccoli
1 clove garlic, minced
1 tablespoon curry powder
1 teaspoon tomato paste
¾ cup chicken or vegetable broth
2 cups cooked brown rice

Season chicken with ginger, basil, paprika or any herb mix. Heat Enhanced Butter Herb Spread in skillet and brown chicken lightly. Add onion, scallion, celery, broccoli and garlic. Cook for 3 minutes. Sprinkle on curry powder and cook another 4 minutes. Stir in tomato paste and broth. Bring to a boil, then reduce heat to medium. Cover skillet and cook chicken until tender. Serve over rice. *Serves 4.*

6

DIET TYPE 3

The No-More-Allergies Diet

A number of years ago, my wife and I decided to go on an "antiallergy" diet. Although we didn't have much weight to lose, we both wanted to be at the peak of health, full of energy and vigor and mentally alert, rather than stressed and fatigued as usual. We had heard reports of how wonderful some people felt after "rotation" dieting: eliminating certain troublesome foods from their diets for a while, then reintroducing them later on in smaller amounts and in a more controlled way.

We started on a very ambitious regimen that allowed us only one food from a particular group or family each day. We could not have the food again for several days, so we always had to plan our meals very carefully. Obviously, the arrangement ruled out leftovers. (What would even the most tasty millet casserole taste like after nearly a week in the refrigerator?) It was also expensive, inconvenient and often downright frustrating. When I woke up each morning, I'd wonder what kinds of meals I could put together from the scant list of "nonallergic" foods arbitrarily assigned to me on a given day. I'd have to hunt for some novel, exotic items in fancy food shops to meet the diet's demand for variety and to avoid repeating the same foods too often. The constant search was exhausting and I could afford only the smallest portions. With so many foods either forbidden or restricted, it was no wonder I lost weight—too much, in fact—and had even less energy than before. (All that meal planning probably took its toll!)

Brown rice happens to be one of my favorite foods. One evening, after four days of abstinence, I found myself looking forward to a big, steaming bowl of it topped with sautéed shrimp and vegetables. But then I realized I had eaten some rice crackers at breakfast that same morning—and so had used up my quota for the day! I felt deprived and cheated; I was determined to find an easier way to diet. If you've already tried an allergy-controlling diet, this may sound like a familiar scenario.

I have since found that, for the vast majority of people, *it's not necessary to go to such lengths to overcome sensitivities to foods and successfully lose weight.* Except in the case of those few individuals with mysterious or obscure patterns of allergy who should be under a physician's close supervision, an overly restrictive plan is impractical and unrealistic; you're unlikely to stay with it long enough to benefit much at all. The No-More-Allergies Diet provides an easier, more flexible way to reach the same goals.

ALLERGY: THE HIDDEN HANDICAP

The notion that you could possibly be allergic to what you eat has attracted widespread attention (and some controversy) lately, but the subject isn't new to medical science. In the early 1930s, Dr. Herbert J. Rinkel, a noted allergist, and his colleagues established a link between intolerances to certain foods and weight problems as well as other troubling symptoms. According to these pioneering doctors and their present-day disciples, particular foods or ingredients may be responsible for skin rashes, breathing difficulties, bloating, migraines, lethargy, nasal congestion, muscle aches and pains, abdominal discomfort and hard-to-control cravings, among other complaints.

Strictly speaking, only about 5 to 10 percent of the population suffers from genuine food allergies (see below). But many other people are sensitive to the chemical compounds in certain foods and experience allergylike symptoms, including mild depression, when they eat them to excess or too often. For example, wheat proteins are chemically similar to some of our brain's own neurotransmitters, known as "endorphins," which are the body's natural painkillers and relaxants. Wheat proteins are broken down by digestion into "exorphins,"* morphinelike compounds that can cause extreme lethargy and drowsiness in some sensitive eaters. Like any addictive drug, they also cause cravings or dependencies that can lead to overweight. "Highs" resulting from wheat, cheese and other foods are all too common!

The point is, regardless of whether you are sensitive or outright allergic to one or more foods, you may have *the same kinds of troubling symptoms*. The textbook distinction may seem meaningless: If you feel below par or acutely uncomfortable after eating any food, it probably matters little to you whether you have a classical allergy or not. You simply want to *feel better*, while staying slim and healthy.

A true food allergy (also known as a fixed allergy) is typically an obvious, sudden or dramatic reaction to a particular item, such as peanuts or shellfish. It may be an immediate attack of migraines or wheezing or an outbreak of hives many hours after a meal. One woman patient I cared for during my training was so allergic to the few bits of nuts in her cookie that she had an anaphylactic shock response; Her throat closed and she was resuscitated in the nick of time in our hospital's emergency room!

* From the Greek *exo*, meaning "out" (here referring to outside the body), and *orphin*, with the same root as the word morphine, meaning a sedating or addicting substance.

As mentioned above, no more than 10 percent of all food reactions fall into this clear-cut allergic category, and the solution is self-evident. Most sufferers know enough to avoid the offending food, and they don't have to overhaul their eating habits to find relief.

Whether it's to pollen, cats, poison ivy, wheat or chocolate, any allergy is an overreaction by the body to something that's tolerated by most people. Normally, your immune system guards you against viruses, bacteria and parasites by producing antibodies that control or kill these invaders. However, if the immune system is somehow defective, it can be indiscriminately aggressive, attacking even harmless or perfectly wholesome substances such as animal dander or dairy foods.

To launch its defense, your body releases high levels of the chemical histamine, as well as antibody proteins issued by the immune system (called IgE and IgG) that can give rise to symptoms anywhere in the body. The gastrointestinal tract is a likely target, and many reactions take the form of nausea, vomiting, gassiness, abdominal pain, constipation or diarrhea. When the histamine and antibody proteins are produced in the blood and lymph, the result is hives, swelling, rashes and itching.

When histamine is released in the lungs, it may constrict the smooth muscles around the bronchial tubes, increase the flow of mucous and make the walls of tiny blood vessels more permeable. As a result, their fluids leak into nearby tissues, causing swelling and blocking of both throat and nasal passages. The familiar "head" complaints of coughing, wheezing, watery eyes and stuffy nose are the final links in this allergic chain of events.

Sometimes, instead of producing hives, rashes or a respiratory attack, your body reacts via your nervous system with mood swings or depression.

There are a host of other food reactions (which I shall refer to simply as "sensitivities") that don't follow the strict allergic histamine/antibody route but result in similar complaints. And some of them don't necessarily make you feel miserable, either, at least not directly: If you're a compulsive overeater or you have strong cravings for a certain item, it's a fair bet that you are food-sensitive. Eating one favorite food or another may give you a powerful but short-lived surge of pleasure. What follows is a period of discomfort, or a kind of withdrawal stage, during which you may feel irritable, tired or intensely hungry until you reach for the same food again to relieve the distress—a common vicious circle. In the case of a persistent craving, the quick fix is so fleeting that you must eat the desired food repeatedly or in large amounts to derive any lasting satisfaction from it—a pattern that is conducive to gaining weight.

Whether or not they're textbook allergies, reactions to the same food can vary widely from person to person. For instance, wheat may bring on pounding headaches in some and hours of intense itching or eczema in others. You may react to a food when you eat it cooked, but not when raw, and vice versa. You can start out with an intolerance to wheat and eventually develop one to other, related foods like barley, rye or oats, all members of the cereal family.

The most common kind of sensitivity results from overexposure to certain foods. You might begin by overindulging in a food every now and then, and soon develop an almost insatiable craving for it. Or you may have no trouble with even large amounts of a single grain or dairy food, but you will have annoying symptoms if you eat more than one kind in the same meal (for example, milk and cheese, or noodles and bread). A good diet that offers sensible portions and enough variety should automatically help prevent you from exceeding your "tolerance threshold" for particular foods.

Both food allergies and sensitivities may show up as delayed reactions (up to two days after you've eaten). They also tend to wax and wane, worsening or only appearing in the presence of a cold, infection or fatigue, or during pollen or hay-fever season. Emotional upsets can provoke a first-time condition or aggravate an existing one.

While any food is a potential allergen, the ones most likely to cause reactions are cow's milk and other dairy foods, wheat, corn, yeast, eggs, nuts, shellfish, soybeans, gluten, some fruits and vegetables, coffee, tea, alcohol and certain food dyes and additives.

How Can Food Allergies Make You Fat?

Consider the paradox: Many people are actually sensitive to their favorite foods, the ones they find hardest to resist and eat frequently or every day. Apparently, they don't feel like themselves when they go for long periods without eating such foods, and that can sabotage their efforts to stay slim. In fact, hidden sensitivities may be a key reason why diets have failed for such people in the past. They simply lose control in the presence of certain foods!

If this pattern describes you, the sanest approach to weight loss and well-being is through an eating plan that can break your addiction to the problem food(s) and interrupt the typical crave/binge/bad feeling/crave and eat again cycle. The No-More-Allergies Diet sets up definite barriers between you and what you eat, thus modifying your behavior and curbing your compulsive habits. You are asked to refrain from reaching for the same kinds of foods repeatedly—a discipline that not only gets you out of a psychological rut, but also promotes efficient weight loss.

In most cases, if you forgo a problem food temporarily, you should be able to tolerate it again in reasonable amounts a short while later, as long as you do so at well-planned intervals.

The secret is to get your timing right! Sometimes, the foods to which you're allergic or sensitive can cause you to retain excess water. Recently, a patient of mine complained that his ears were ringing all the time. He was taking antibiotics for recurrent bouts of bronchitis, and I suspected that he might have developed an intestinal overgrowth of yeast (see page 182). He also craved sugar and freshly baked breads, another clue that he could be allergic to yeast. Sure enough, when I put him on a yeast-free diet plus medications that eradicated intestinal yeast, his ear symptoms disappeared. Remarkably, he also started losing weight at the rate of two pounds a day, for a total of eighteen pounds in nine days! Histamines released throughout his body in response to yeast had provoked widespread water retention. An undiagnosed food sensitivity may well be blocking your way to a slimmer body, particularly if you feel bloated and puffy all the time.

Short of reacting with immediate, obvious symptoms, how can you tell whether or not you're intolerant of certain foods? Blood and skin tests are far from conclusive when it comes to detecting most food allergies, let alone other kinds of food sensitivities. The only sure way to tell is to eliminate all the prime suspects from your diet for a few weeks, and note how you feel. Then start reintroducing them one at a time, again keeping track of your responses. By clearing your diet of all potential problem foods and then adding them back individually, you should be able to isolate the source(s) of your distress.

THE NO-MORE-ALLERGIES ELIMINATION DIET

For ten days, this diet will help you steer clear of all the leading problem foods: dairy foods, wheat, corn, sugar, yeast, eggs, nuts, shellfish, coffee, tea, alcohol, gluten, some fruits and vegetables, and preservatives (e.g., BHT, BHA, nitrites, sulfites).

During this time, by simply eliminating all the items in the groups listed below you will automatically rule out the "forbidden" foods.

MEAT: Do not eat prepared meat loaf, sausage, commercial breaded fish or meat patties, cured bacon or ham, hot dogs, cold cuts, luncheon meats, meats fried in cracker crumbs or flour, or meat gravies.

VEGETABLES: Eliminate corn on the cob, canned and frozen corn, tomatoes, potatoes, eggplants, mushrooms, truffles, pickles and sauerkraut.

CEREALS, GRAINS, PASTAS, BREADS: Avoid all hot and cold cereals except those made from brown rice, millet or amaranth (available in health-food stores), and all pastas except those made from pure Jerusalem artichoke, rice or soy flour; also, eat no pretzels, melba toast, bread crumbs or croutons, and only breads or crackers baked with rice or soy flour.

FRUITS: Do not eat citrus fruits.

COOKING OILS: Eliminate corn, cottonseed, peanut and vegetable oils.

DAIRY PRODUCTS: Avoid cow's milk (whole or skim); cheese; buttermilk; ice cream; sherbet; yogurt; butter; margarine; nondairy creamers; canned or cream-based soups, sauces and gravies; cocoa mixes; pancakes; waffles; puddings and baking mixes. Check labels on candies, cookies and breads to make sure no dairy ingredients are present.

EGGS: Do not eat cakes, cookies and other bakery products made with eggs; egg noodles, mayonnaise, salad dressings; hollandaise sauce, malted cocoa drinks, marshmallows, custards, meringues and soufflés. Note: Wines are often cleared with egg whites and many prepared foods contain dried or powdered eggs.

YEAST: Avoid brewer's, baker's and torula yeast, biscuits, vinegars, catsup, commercial soy sauce, horseradish, canned or frozen citrus juices and bouillon cubes (except the yeast-free kind).

SUGAR: Stay away from candies, cookies, cakes, pastries, pies, jams, jellies, gelatin desserts, foods with added sugars (glucose, sucrose, dextrose, maltose, maltodextrin, fructose), corn syrup and chocolate.

NUTS: Avoid nuts and nut butters; seeds like pumpkin, sesame and sunflower are okay.

SEAFOOD: Eat no shellfish.

BEVERAGES: Abstain from all alcoholic drinks, regular tea and coffee, caffeinated or decaffeinated (use herbal teas instead).

CONDIMENTS, SPICES, ADDITIVES: Avoid baking powder (except if made without wheat or corn), sulfates, sulfites, nitrates, nitrites, BHT, food colorings and MSG.

It's no coincidence that most of the foods on the forbidden list are highly processed—and fattening. Allergies aside, ruling out these high-calorie offenders for a week or more is an excellent weight-loss strategy. Stick to whole, fresh, simple foods. The boxed, canned and bottled kinds are most likely to add extra pounds *and* cause troubling symptoms.

Diet Type 3 is a sample one-week menu plan eliminating all the potential food allergens cited above and highlighting fresh, whole, unprocessed foods. The diet's high-fiber complex carbohydrates release energy gradually; unlike simple sugars and fats, which provide a "quick fix," such foods prevent the abrupt peaks and valleys in both appetite and energy that often lead to destructive cravings and binges in the first place. They are also naturally satisfying and rich in vitamins and minerals. In many cases, you can eat as much as you want of the desirable foods; this diet places less emphasis on strict portion control than many comparable ones. Also, since allergies are sometimes responsible for bloating and swelling resulting from fluid retention, the elimination strategy should cause the extra unflattering water weight to disappear as well.

While this eating plan is primarily aimed at those with suspected food sensitivities, even if you are free of such problems you may find the diet an extremely effective weight-loss tool.

WHAT NEXT?

If you feel significantly better after ten days, it's time to re-challenge yourself with foods to discover which ones are giving you trouble. The No-More-Allergies Elimination Diet is the base to which you'll add variety in a strategic way as you put back the foods eliminated during week one. Restore one category of food from the original "scratch" list to your diet every 48 hours. (You need to wait this long between reintroduced foods since some allergic or sensitivity reactions might be delayed.)

Add each food in its simplest form. Start with pure milk products: milk, cream or cottage cheese instead of ice cream, which contains eggs. Then try pure wheat. Eat cream of wheat cereal or yeastless soda crackers (instead of whole wheat bread, which contains yeast and sometimes eggs). Next add eggs, then pure corn, followed by the other foods one by one.

If you experience any reactions, stop eating the food and wait until your symptoms subside. Then retest the suspected item. Once you identify which reintroduced foods trouble you most, remove them from your diet for a whole month, then try to eat them once every five days on a rotating basis. Keep in mind that this system does not work for serious, fixed food allergies; adding back nuts or seafood to a menu even after months of avoidance won't help if you have a strong histamine/antibody reaction to them, like my woman patient who was near death from anaphylactic shock.

Of course, you may already know to which foods you're sensitive—and none may have appeared on the original list. If you have a chronic craving for chicken or feel queasy after eating onions, for example, eliminate those items and then reintroduce them a week later as described above. Remember, the aim of this diet is to give you a means of handling *any* food sensitivities while you control your weight.

As we've seen, an allergy or sensitivity generally results from overexposure to foods, or the tendency to eat them too

WATCH OUT FOR HIDDEN INGREDIENTS!

If you're sensitive to corn, you might not think of eliminating a wheat breakfast cereal from your diet unless you read the label carefully and discover that one of its many ingredients is corn syrup. It's the not-so-obvious sources of allergens found often in highly processed foods that pose the greatest nuisance and can easily be overlooked in products with a well-padded label.

If you can't tolerate corn, be aware that it's found in places you'd never think of, such as salad dressings, sandwich spreads, certain ice creams, canned creamed soups, cakes, candies, catsup, puffed-rice cereals, syrup and cured bacon. Wheat is used as a binder in prepared foods and soups, hot dogs, sausages, some ice creams and most rye breads. Many people are sensitive to cottonseed oil, which is used in most bottled salad dressings, margarines, potato chips and doughnuts. Those who react to soybeans must avoid bakery products, soy and Worcestershire sauce, sausages, cold cuts, Crisco oil and processed cheeses. Hot dogs, even the 100 percent beef kind, contain cereal, preservatives and filler.

Remember, the less complicated and tampered with the foods you eat are, the less likely that you'll be troubled by any "hidden" ingredients.

often, rather than from sporadic and reasonable consumption. If you react to one or more foods, you most likely have a tolerance threshold; by rotating or eating foods at well-timed intervals, you can keep them from ever reaching this critical point. That means you can continue to enjoy favorite or nutritionally important foods instead of banning them entirely.

Two exceptions to this rule may be wheat and milk. Some people can't have even small amounts of them infrequently without experiencing distress. All you're asked to do is broaden your diet, stretch your imagination and add versatility to your previously one-track-minded menus so you won't end up overdepending on any one food. Since you will break the pattern that promotes out-of-control cravings, you should lose weight steadily, too.

Note: The emphasis on unprocessed, low-fat foods can also help strengthen your body's resistance to degenerative and contagious diseases. And if you already react to airborne allergens—dust, pollen, animal dander, molds, chemicals and the like—you may find you're better able to tolerate them while following this diet.

To summarize:

STEP I:

Eliminate

Follow elimination diet for ten days to two weeks. If you feel better (have fewer cravings, less severe symptoms, loss of water weight), go on to Step II.

STEP II:

Test

Methodically test all eliminated foods while continuing the basic elimination diet. Reinstate each eliminated food for 48 hours, noting symptoms on the Progress Calendar (see page 188).

STEP III:

Add Back

Eliminate symptom-producing foods for *one full month*. During this time, all other foods can be added back except those on the Worst-Offender List (wheat, corn, dairy, eggs, nuts), which are to be eaten on a five-day rotation basis only.

STEP IV:

Add Back

After one month, try adding back symptom-producing foods on a five-day rotation basis. Eliminate them if you react unfavorably; if you tolerate them well, you may continue to eat them *once every five days*. Foods on the Worst-Offender List should be on a five-day rotation *permanently*. Your ongoing No-More-Allergies Diet might look like this if you found you were sensitive, say, to citrus fruits and barley, but tolerated them on a rotation basis, and always reacted to shellfish, no matter how infrequently you ate it.

Mon.	*Tues.*	*Wed.*	*Thur.*	*Fri.*	*Sat.*	*Sun*	*Mon.*	*Tues.*	*Wed.*
citrus wheat	corn	dairy	barley eggs	nuts	citrus wheat	corn	dairy	barley eggs	nuts

WORST-OFFENDER LIST:

The following foods should be rotated every five days no matter what:

- wheat
- corn
- milk/dairy products
- eggs
- nuts

A FRESH START

Have you ever noticed that when you first begin a new diet—any diet—you feel great, refreshed, renewed, full of energy? Think about it. At the outset, almost any eating plan acts like the No-More-Allergies Diet because it gets you to eat differently than you did before, shaking you free of some unhealthy habits. But because it doesn't *rotate* meals in a methodical way, you may soon find yourself craving and overeating the "new" foods, too.

FOOD ALLERGY/SENSITIVITY: WHAT ARE THE SYMPTOMS?

Wheat or Gluten
Eczema
Cramps
Bloating
Gas
Diarrhea
Colitis
Asthma
Hay fever
Headaches
Depression

Milk
Stuffy or runny nose
Asthma
Ear infection
Rashes
Vomiting
Bloating
Stomach pains, gassiness, indigestion
Diarrhea
Leg aches
Bed-wetting (children)

Eggs
Gall bladder attacks
Gastritis
Indigestion
Migraines
Acne
Diarrhea
Eczema

Corn
Migraines
Hives
Gastritis
Colitis
Rhinitis
Asthma

Yeast
Lack of concentration
Vaginitis
Urinary frequency
Abdominal bloating
Sinusitis
Sore throats
Headaches
Constipation/diarrhea
Fatigue
Anxiety, depression
Aching muscles
Menstrual irregularities

Nightshade Vegetables
Mouth ulcers
Arthritic joints
Depression

Fruits
Drowsiness
Mouth Ulcers
Nasal congestion
Abdominal bloating
Asthma

Coffee, Tea	**Chocolate**	**Nuts**
Arthritis	Migraines	Mouth Ulcers
Gall bladder	Diarrhea	Acne
attacks	Acne	Herpes flare-ups
Headache	Behavioral	Hives
Palpitations	problems	
Urinary frequency	Heartburn	
Diarrhea		

MILK: ALLERGY OR LACTOSE INTOLERANCE?

Some people are unable to digest lactose, or milk sugar, especially as they age. Blacks, Hispanics, Orientals, Indians and many Mediterranean peoples often lose the milk-digesting enzyme, lactase, early in childhood; however, northern and western Europeans tend to lose it much later in life, if at all. Apparently, the genes that are required to digest lactose have been preserved over the generations in northern and western Europe, where milk is a dietary staple. This is also the case in some non-Caucasian areas such as central Asia, where the population relies heavily on milk from their local livestock.

Symptoms of lactose intolerance include stomach and intestinal upset, diarrhea and bloating after a meal of milk or ice cream. To find out whether you're affected, your doctor can perform a simple test by giving you a small amount of pure lactose. If your own blood sugar level doesn't rise within minutes, you haven't absorbed any of the milk sugar —which means your body lacks the enzyme needed to handle it. Alternatively, the recently developed "hydrogen breath test" can be performed.

For those deficient in the milk-digesting lactase, Lactaid low-fat (1 percent) milk, slightly sweeter than the regular kind, contains the missing enzyme. Liquid Lactaid, available from pharmacies, can be added to milk when you're traveling. Yogurt, kefir and some cheeses pose no problem since they're cultured milk products, in which the natural process of fermentation has already "digested" much of the lactose.

Cheddar and Cheshire cheese are very low in lactose, while aged Edam and Gouda contain none at all. Cottage cheese has 86 percent less than regular milk.

If you are truly allergic to milk, however, you will probably be sensitive to cheese and yogurt as well since this allergy is usually an overreaction to milk *protein.* Especially when an allergic person's digestive tract cannot take apart the large milk protein molecules, casein and beta-lactoglobulin, these enter the bloodstream unchanged, causing a reaction. Goat's milk has a different protein, and thus is usually less allergenic. Heating or evaporating the milk can help break the proteins down. You might also tolerate whole milk, butter and cheese better than skim or low-fat milk, since fat slows down protein absorption, giving the body more time to adjust to the oversized molecules.

However, another kind of milk intolerance involves fat malabsorption, making you sensitive to all fats, including the ones found in anything *but* skim-milk dairy foods. Obviously, foods like sour cream, rich ice cream and heavy cream would trigger the strongest reactions. It's not uncommon for people to be allergic *and* lactose intolerant, since allergy may cause an inflammation of the intestinal tract and compromise the ability to digest lactose. Lactase activity may also shut down temporarily in the presence of a stomach virus or bacterial infection or after taking antibiotics.

IS THERE A YEAST CONNECTION?

You may have heard a lot about yeast infections lately, as these prolific organisms are key players in a surprising number of bodily complaints. Some allergists believe that diets high in refined, simple carbohydrates along with an overreliance on antibiotics have resulted in a near epidemic of undiagnosed and untreated infections by a fungus known as *candida albicans,* a substance similar to the yeast used in making bread and beer.

While the diagnosis remains questionable to many orthodox medical practitioners, candida has been labeled by others as responsible for a wide variety of ills, including vaginitis, chronic fatigue, bloating, constipation, diarrhea, aching muscles, lethargy, headaches, menstrual and bladder irregularities, even anxiety and depression. Yeast normally resides inside the gastrointestinal tract and other moist, warm areas like the mouth, throat, vagina and rectum. Normally, a healthy immune system keeps the growth under control. However, when our bodily defenses are weakened by an illness, for example, or when the "friendly" bacteria in our small and large intestines are diminished by the use of certain drugs, yeast can multiply freely—enough to cause physical and psychological symptoms. Women are more commonly afflicted than men, possibly because estrogen favors the growth of yeast.

The risk factors that predispose someone to candida include the following:

- a history of taking antibiotics, particularly those of the tetracycline family
- prolonged illness, especially one that compromises the immune system, such as AIDS
- undernutrition
- chemotherapy or irradiation
- a history of taking cortisone (corticosteroids)
- a diet high in sweets, fruits and juices
- multiple pregnancies
- use of birth control pills or hormone replacement
- diabetes
- alcoholism or any excessive use of alcohol

To check for candida, a physician may take fungus cultures from several likely target organs; a large number of organisms suggests that the yeast is out of hand throughout the body, causing mischief. Sometimes, a physician may suggest a trial of treatment if he or she suspects candida is present; the patient is monitored for any signs of symptom relief to confirm the diagnosis.

Candida is not a new disease. Medical documents prove that it has been around for at least several centuries. However, it's considered more prevalent today because of the widespread use of the predisposing drugs mentioned above as well as the refinements in diet that have made it easier to overindulge in highly sweetened, nutritionally deficient foods.

CONFRONTING CANDIDA

Just as the origins of this condition are multiple, so are the means of attacking it. Live-culture yogurt and kefir (containing lactobacillus acidophilus) can restore the growth of favorable intestinal bacteria that help put the reins on candida activity. Since yeasts thrive on sweets, avoid any excess of them in your diet. Eliminate or cut way down on white and brown sugar, honey, maple and corn syrup, molasses, baked goods and presweetened breakfast cereals as well as milk, molded cheeses like Blue and Roquefort, fruit (especially the dried kind and juices) and alcohol. A highly nutritious diet will keep your immune system functioning at peak level; eat plenty of fresh (nonstarchy) vegetables, moderate amounts of whole grains (yeast-free whenever possible), seafood, poultry, lean meats, plain low-fat yogurt or kefir, seeds and low-fat nuts. When symptoms subside you can add some low-sugar fruits, such as apples and pears. Fresh garlic and onion are both natural fungus-fighters, so try cooking with these whenever possible. If you are trying to lose weight and are consuming less than 1,600 calories a day, a good (yeast-free) multivitamin/mineral supplement will ensure that you receive at least the RDAs for all important nutrients. Other doctor-supervised approaches include taking lactobacillus acidophilus tablets, supplements of the B complex and vitamin C and, for stubborn cases, prescription antifungal medications such as Nystatin or Nizoral.

Note: Allergy and sensitivity to foods and chemicals are often associated with susceptibility to candida infections.

THE FOOD-ALLERGY CONTROVERSY

Most physicians recognize only obvious, "fixed" allergies—the explosive, hypersensitive reactions, such as an outbreak of hives after eating a single strawberry, or a series of throat-constricting wheezes following a meal of seafood or nuts. But these dramatic examples are far less common than the more subtle kinds of sensitivities that result from repeated exposure to certain foods or from an unrecognized dependency on them.

Why is the idea of food allergy often dismissed or overlooked? To put it simply, many physicians are not that well-informed about nutrition, as most medical schools offer little or no formal training in the subject. Typically, physicians have not had more than a few hours of instruction on the subject, and they are trained to offer specific prescriptions for medical solutions to illnesses, rather than to help patients by altering their diets or lifestyles. Going on a diet that first identifies and then controls sensitivities to foods is not a quick fix or a prescription, but an exploratory and sometimes time-consuming process. It's definitely worth the effort, but it's not popular in an age when therapy is often dispensed in tablet form.

Another problem is that the evidence for food sensitivities is considered too subjective compared with that for inhalant allergies, such as those to dust, mold, animals and plants. Unlike the latter, a number of food allergies cannot be verified by blood and/or skin tests, and so proof frequently depends on a patient's personal impressions. Many physicians also dispute the notion that sensitivities to foods can possibly produce such "emotional" symptoms as depression or irritability.

On the other hand, nutrition-oriented physicians sometimes attribute *too many* symptoms to food and overlook other causes or influences—to the extent that they invite their colleagues' disbelief. Food allergy is not a rampant threat, nor does its elimination promise a cure for killer dis-

KEEPING A FOOD DIARY

To help give yourself as well as your doctor an accurate account of your response to certain foods, keep a daily food log or diary to record what and how much you eat every day, along with how you feel and when symptoms arise. It's best not to depend on memory, so jot this information down in a small, portable notebook. The more detailed your "evidence," the more quickly you will be able to solve your case. Also, consider rating your responses on a scale from "mild" to "severe."

Since so much eating is automatic, the diary is also a strategic weight-loss aid that can work on any diet (see also Chapter 9). By recording how you feel, you will be able to see the emotional states that encourage you to nosh. Once you observe how much you eat or how often, it should be easier to modify your behavior. "Challenge Foods" are the foods you will introduce one at a time after having eliminated them from your diet temporarily.

The Elimination Diet Progress Calendar on page 188 has been indispensable for many of my patients in their search for troublemaking foods and habits.

One way to start rounding up leading food suspects is to mark down the days when you feel normal or terrific and those when you don't, and note what you have eaten on each day. Whatever foods are not common to *both* lists might well be giving you a problem.

eases such as cancer or AIDS. I think the truth definitely lies somewhere in between—food reactions account for a fair share of complaints, both physical and emotional, for which no other medical origin can be found. In the future, new technology should make it easier to accurately identify and measure these sensitivities.

ALLERGIES MAKE YOU FAT

If people tended to overeat because of an allergy to, say, cucumbers or zucchini, they wouldn't have to worry about gaining weight. Unfortunately, most addictive allergies are to foods that can be fattening if eaten to excess. Wheat, eggs, milk, corn and yeast are often prime ingredients in high-fat, calorie-loaded foods. Alas, those with a strong allergic craving for wheat more frequently binge on refined foods like pastries and cakes than on a more healthful, lower-calorie form like stone-ground whole-wheat bread!

Meanwhile, however, doctors do have to rely largely on what their patients tell them. Keeping a detailed food diary (see page 186) and following the directions given for the No-More-Allergies-Diet can provide an accurate account of symptoms. (In fact, this is the essence of a good, thorough medical history. Without a patient's full disclosure, a doctor's ability to treat *any* condition can be seriously compromised.)

LACTOSE-FREE CHEESES

Brick
Camembert
Cheddar
Edam
Provolone
Swiss
Pasteurized Process American Cheese

ELIMINATION DIET PROGRESS CALENDAR

	BREAKFAST	LUNCH	DINNER	SNACK	SYMPTOMS
DAY # ___ OF DIET Date: _____ Foods eliminated: _____ Challenge foods: _____ *Wt. _____					
DAY # ___ OF DIET Date: _____ Foods eliminated: _____ Challenge foods: _____ Wt. _____					
DAY # ___ OF DIET Date: _____ Foods eliminated: _____ Challenge foods: _____ Wt. _____					
DAY # ___ OF DIET Date: _____ Foods eliminated: _____ Challenge foods: _____ Wt. _____					
DAY # ___ OF DIET Date: _____ Foods eliminated: _____ Challenge foods: _____ Wt. _____					
DAY # ___ OF DIET Date: _____ Foods eliminated: _____ Challenge foods: _____ Wt. _____					
DAY # ___ OF DIET Date: _____ Foods eliminated: _____ Challenge foods: _____ Wt. _____					

* Weight first thing in the morning (after voiding)

One way for physicians to identify food allergies more objectively would be to give patients harmless placebos and unmarked capsules containing various foods, thus allowing them to separate genuine reactions from imagined or exaggerated ones. This would be a responsible and open-minded approach that might earn the respect of the wider medical community until more scientific tests are devised.

SAMPLE MENUS

Recipes are provided for all dishes marked with an asterisk (*). To find recipes that appear in other sections, consult the Index at the back of this book.

Beverages for all meals: herbal tea, soy milk, seltzer, plain or sparkling mineral water, fresh vegetable juices or filtered tap water.

DAY 1:

Breakfast

Rice cream cereal

Cooked Apple*

Lunch

Two-Bean Salad*

Millet with Cauliflower and Onions*

Dinner

Oriental Stir-Fry*

Rice with Carrots and Onions*

Snacks

Rice cakes

Local fruit: apples, grapes, pears

DAY 2:

Breakfast

Rice Bread with Apple Butter*

Lunch

Sardines and Broccoli with Garlic*

Dinner

Rice and Lentil Loaf with No-Allergy Mustard Topping*

Steamed kale

Baked sweet potato

Snacks

Rice cakes

Local fruit: apples, grapes, pears

DAY 3:

Breakfast

Puffed millet

Soy milk (plain) with rice syrup

Lunch
Shredded Vegetables with Lean Hamburger*

Salad

Zucchini Squash*

Dinner
Vegetable Seed Loaf*

Sautéed Broccoli and Cauliflower*

Snacks
Rice cakes

Local fruit: apples, grapes, pears

DAY 4:

Breakfast
Quinoa Pudding* with cooked pears

Lunch
Holiday Sweet Potatoes with Flaked Salmon*

Romaine, cucumber and carrot salad with Herbal Nonallergenic Dressing*

Dinner
Lentil Soup with Escarole and Carrots*

Fluffy Millet-Amaranth Soufflé*

Ginger-Glazed Carrots*

Snacks

Rice cakes

Local fruit: apples, grapes, pears

DAY 5:

Breakfast

Rice cakes with natural fruit conserves

Lunch

Super Rice-Noodle Tofu*

Salad

Peas

Dinner

Broccoli Soup*

No-Tomato Sauce on Rice Pasta*

Steamed cauliflower

Snacks

Rice cakes

Local fruit: apples, grapes, pears

DAY 6:

Breakfast

Cooked amaranth with sliced peaches

Lunch

Chicken Cubes with Onions and Vegetables*

String Beans*

Dinner

Lima Beans and Quinoa*

Salad

Snacks

Rice cakes

Local fruit: apples, grapes, pears

DAY 7:

Breakfast

Puffed brown rice cereal with raisins and cinnamon

Soy milk

Lunch

Chinese Tuna Salad*

Dinner

Stuffed Cornish Hen*

Steamed collards

Snacks

Rice cakes

Local fruit: apples, grapes, pears

▬▬▬▬▬ ■ ▬▬▬▬▬

FIVE EASY PIECES

Satisfying, nutritious, portable lunch/dinner alternatives that you can prepare with a minimum of fuss and effort. Each makes one individual portion.

1. *Avocado spread*

   Mix ½ mashed avocado, 2–3 finely sliced radishes, 1 teaspoon chopped toasted sunflower seeds and ¼ onion, finely chopped. Spread on rice cracker and top with alfalfa sprouts.

2. *Sesame chicken*

   Slice 3-ounce cooked skinless chicken breast into thin strips. Mix with 1 teaspoon toasted sesame seeds, ¼ cup finely diced celery and 1 teaspoon low-sodium soy sauce. Serve garnished with salad fixings.

3. *Sweet tuna salad*

   Fork-blend one 3½-ounce individual can water-packed tuna with 2 tablespoons diced pineapple, ½ chopped kiwi, and a dash of cinnamon. Serve on rice crackers.

4. *Sesame rice salad*

   Dilute 1 teaspoon tahini (sesame butter) with 1 tablespoon water. Add 1 teaspoon dark sesame oil, 1 teaspoon low-sodium soy sauce and a pinch of garlic powder. Blend 1 cup leftover brown rice with chopped romaine lettuce, radishes, scallions, and red peppers. Top with sesame dressing and toss well.

5. *Tropical sweet potato salad*

   Slice ½ cooked sweet potato into chunks. Mix with ½ Granny Smith apple, finely diced; ¼ ripe banana, mashed; and 1 teaspoon toasted sunflower seeds. Serve on bed of romaine lettuce.

■

RECIPES

Cooked apple   *1st Day Breakfast*

1 apple
Pinch of cinnamon
Few drops of water

Wash apple and peel if desired. Cut out core and seeds; slice into eighths. Cook in small pot over low heat with water and cinnamon for approximately 10–12 minutes. Serve with cooked cereals. *Serves 1.*

Two-bean salad   *1st Day Lunch*

1 cup dried lima beans
4 cups water
½ carrot
½ onion
3 sprigs fresh parsley
½ teaspoon sea salt
½–1 cup fresh sliced string beans
1 tablespoon chives
Fresh basil
1 scallion
1–2 tablespoons olive oil
2 tablespoons vinegar (distilled is free of common allergens)

Wash beans, place in water and bring to a boil. Simmer for 2 minutes; then cover, turn off heat and let sit for 2 hours. Add carrot, onion and 1 parsley sprig, and simmer for 1 hour. Add salt ½ hour before beans are fully cooked. Remove carrot, onion and parsley and discard. Drain beans and allow to cool. Steam string beans until tender, approximately 7 minutes.

Chop chives, basil, 2 parsley sprigs and scallion together. In a large bowl combine 1½ cups cooked lima beans, the string beans and herbs. Toss with oil and vinegar. Mix well with a wooden spoon. *Serves 2.*

Millet with cauliflower and onions   1st Day Lunch

1½ cups cooked millet
½ cup chopped steamed cauliflower florets
⅓ cup steamed onions
½ teaspoon basil
1 tablespoon soy oil
⅓ teaspoon salt

Combine all ingredients and mix well. Serve hot. *Serves 2.*

Oriental stir-fry   1st Day Dinner

2 tablespoons olive oil
4 celery stalks, chopped
½ cauliflower, sliced thin
½ cup sliced steamed brussels sprouts
6 onions, chopped
1 zucchini, sliced thin
1 green pepper, cut in strips
½ teaspoon salt
1 teaspoon Sesame Salt*
¼ teaspoon grated ginger
¼ teaspoon marjoram
1 tablespoon water

Heat oil in wok. Sauté vegetables in oil for 5 minutes, stirring frequently. Add seasonings and water, cover and simmer for 2 minutes more. *Serves 4.*

*Sesame Salt:
1 cup roasted sesame seeds
2 teaspoons sea salt

Grind seeds until half crushed in a mortar or suribachi (Japanese mortar). Add salt; grind well into the seeds. *Yield: ½ cup Sesame Salt*

Rice with carrots and onions   1st Day Dinner

½ cup chopped steamed carrots
⅓ cup chopped onion
Pinch of thyme
½ tablespoon sesame oil
1 cup cooked brown, converted or basmati rice

Sauté carrots, onion and thyme in oil until tender. Combine with cooked rice; mix well. Serve hot. *Serves 2.*

Rice bread with apple butter   2nd Day Breakfast

1 cup rice flour
4 teaspoons Arrowroot Baking Powder (see p. 109)
½ teaspoon salt
1 tablespoon rice syrup
¾ cup water
2 tablespoons oil

Preheat oven to 350 degrees. Sift all dry ingredients. Add the rice syrup, water and oil. Bake in a loaf pan for 50 minutes. Let bread cool, slice and spread with apple butter. *Serves 3.*

Sardines and broccoli with garlic   2nd Day Lunch

6 ounces water-packed sardines

Broccoli with Garlic:
¼ head broccoli
1–2 cloves garlic, peeled and sliced or crushed
Dash of olive oil
Salt and pepper to taste

Wash broccoli; break apart florets and chop stems (use only florets if desired). Steam in stainless steel steamer basket for approximately 3 minutes or until desired tenderness is reached. Sauté garlic in olive oil over low heat; watch that it doesn't get too hot. When garlic's aroma is released, turn off heat. Toss over steamed broccoli; add salt and pepper to taste. May be served hot or chilled. *Serves 1.*

Rice and lentil loaf with
no-allergy mustard topping   2nd Day Dinner

¾ cup chopped onion
2 tablespoons water
1 tablespoon olive oil
2 cups cooked lentils
½ cup cooked brown rice
¼ cup texturized vegetable protein (TVP)
½ cup crushed rice crackers
¾ cup soy milk
4 cloves garlic, finely chopped
½ teaspoon salt
¼ teaspoon sage
¼ teaspoon marjoram
1 teaspoon onion powder
¼ teaspoon garlic powder

Preheat oven to 350 degrees. Sauté onion in water and oil. Mix all ingredients well and bake in an oiled loaf pan for 1 hour. *Serves 4.*

No-Allergy Mustard Topping:
3 tablespoons olive oil
2 tablespoons rice flour
½ teaspoon dry mustard
1 cup vegetable, poultry or beef broth
1 tablespoon apple juice

Heat olive oil and stir in flour and mustard. Slowly add broth and apple juice, stirring constantly.

Shredded vegetables with lean hamburger   3rd Day Lunch

4 ounces lean ground beef, (chuck, eye round, bottom round, etc.)
1 onion, chopped
½ cup shredded cabbage
1½ tablespoons olive oil
1 parsnip, shredded
1 clove garlic, minced
¼ teaspoon oregano
¼ teaspoon sage
¼ teaspoon marjoram

Shape beef into patty and cook on top of stove at medium heat, or broil or barbecue if desired. Cut into cubes. Sauté onion and cabbage with oil in skillet, stirring constantly, for 5 minutes. Reduce heat and continue cooking for 5 minutes more. Add parsnip and garlic and sauté 5 minutes. Add seasonings and cubed beef to vegetable mixture and stir well. Cook 3 minutes longer. *Serves 2.*

Zucchini squash *3rd Day Lunch*

1 zucchini
Dash of olive oil
1–2 cloves fresh garlic, crushed
Salt and pepper to taste

Wash zucchini and slice into thin rounds. Sauté in skillet
with oil and garlic. Add salt and pepper to taste. Zucchini
may also be steamed until tender in stainless steel steamer
basket. *Serves 2.*

Vegetable seed loaf *3rd Day Dinner*

⅔ cup cubed carrot
½ onion
1 cup cubed zucchini
½ cup toasted sesame seeds
½ cup sunflower seeds
½ cup pumpkin seeds
½ cup celery, finely chopped
½ teaspoon basil
1 teaspoon tarragon
½ teaspoon powdered sage
2½ tablespoons arrowroot flour
⅔ teaspoon salt
2 tablespoons sesame oil

Preheat oven to 375 degrees. Place carrot, onion and zucchini
in stainless steel steamer basket and steam until tender.
Meanwhile, grind seeds in blender or food processor until
mealy. Place in large bowl. Mince cooked onion, then add
all vegetables to seed mixture. Grind to soft consistency. Add
remaining ingredients and mix well. Spread evenly in
greased loaf or casserole pan, and bake for approximately 20
minutes. *Serves 4.*

Sautéed broccoli and cauliflower   *3rd Day Dinner*

1 teaspoon sesame oil
½ cup chopped broccoli florets
½ cup cauliflower florets
Few drops of tamari (soy) sauce (optional)
2 teaspoons water (optional)

Heat oil in wok. Add vegetables and toss lightly. Add tamari, if desired, and cover. Do not use high heat. Add water if vegetables begin to stick. Cook approximately 7–10 minutes or until desired consistency is reached. Serve immediately. *Serves 2.*

Quinoa pudding   *4th Day Breakfast*

1 cup cooked quinoa (grain available from health-food store)
1 pear, cubed
2 tablespoons rice syrup
¼ teaspoon cinnamon

Combine all ingredients. Serve hot. *Serves 1.*

Holiday sweet potatoes with flaked salmon   *4th Day Lunch*

Baked Salmon:
6 ounces fresh salmon
Few drops of lemon juice
Few drops of water
Dill, fresh or dried
Parsley, fresh or dried
Pepper

Preheat oven to 375 degrees. Place salmon in baking dish with lemon and water. Sprinkle with dill and parsley. Bake until fish is flaky. Pepper to taste. Flake fish and set aside.

6 tablespoons tapioca flour
6 tablespoons water
1 teaspoon baking powder
1 tablespoon safflower oil
1 cup soy milk
2 cups cooked, mashed sweet potatoes
6 ounces baked salmon, flaked
½ cup toasted sunflower seeds
1½ teaspoons cinnamon
¼ teaspoon nutmeg
½ teaspoon allspice
½ teaspoon cloves
1 tablespoon frozen apple-juice concentrate, thawed

Preheat oven to 325 degrees. Combine tapioca and water and cook, stirring until mixture thickens. Add baking powder and oil. Remove from heat. Beat soy milk into mixture. Stir into mashed sweet potatoes and blend thoroughly. Stir in salmon flakes, sunflower seeds, spices and apple-juice concentrate. Place mixture in oiled casserole dish and bake for 20 minutes. *Serves 3.*

Herbal nonallergenic dressing   4th Day Lunch

⅓ cup olive oil
2 teaspoons finely chopped onions
2 teaspoons chopped chives
3 tablespoons apple juice
¼ teaspoon marjoram
¼ teaspoon celery seed
2 sprigs fresh parsley

Blend in a blender and refrigerate. *Yield: ½ cup.*

Lentil soup with escarole and carrots   4th Day Dinner

½ pound lentils
6 cups water

2 carrots, diced small
2 cloves garlic, crushed
Dash of extra-virgin olive oil
1 cup escarole, washed and cut into small pieces
Salt and pepper to taste
Tamari (soy) sauce (optional)

Wash lentils and remove stones. Bring water to a boil, add lentils and cook for 30 minutes or until tender. Add remaining ingredients to lentils and simmer covered until carrots are tender. Add salt and pepper and/or tamari to taste. Serve hot. *Serves 6.*

Fluffy millet-amaranth soufflé   *4th Day Dinner*

½ cup amaranth
1½ cups millet
2 ears of corn (kernels only)
½ cup diced carrots
½ cup diced bok choy
½ cup diced celery
3 scallions, chopped
½ cup diced onions
¼ cup diced cauliflower
3 cups water
¼ teaspoon ground ginger
¼ teaspoon sage
¼ teaspoon basil
Pinch of salt
1 tablespoon chopped parsley
Sesame Salt (see page 197) (optional)

Wash amaranth and millet separately. Roast millet in frying pan for a few minutes until golden. Place millet, amaranth and vegetables in pressure cooker. Add water and seasonings. Cover pressure cooker and place on medium-high heat until pressure rises. Reduce heat to low and cook 15 minutes.

Remove from heat and let pressure come down. Serve topped with parsley. Sesame Salt is optional for taste. *Serves 4.*

Ginger-glazed carrots   *4th Day Dinner*

4 carrots
Dash of sesame oil
⅛ teaspoon ground ginger
2 teaspoons rice syrup
Fresh chopped mint

Scrub carrots; peel if not organically grown. Steam in stainless steel steamer basket until almost tender. Heat oil, ginger and rice syrup in skillet. Add carrots and coat with sauce. Cook slowly over low heat for another minute or so, until carrots are tender. Garnish with chopped mint. *Serves 2.*

Super rice-noodle tofu   *5th Day Lunch*

2 cups rice noodles
1 onion, chopped
½ cup sunflower seeds
2 tablespoons sunflower oil
1 tablespoon kuzu or arrowroot
½ cup water
1 cup finely cubed tofu
½ teaspoon salt
1 teaspoon Sesame Salt (see page 197)
1 teaspoon grated ginger
¼ teaspoon thyme
½ teaspoon rosemary
¼ teaspoon paprika
Pinch of cayenne
No-Tomato Sauce for topping (see page 206)

Preheat oven to 325 degrees. Cook noodles, drain and rinse with cold water. Sauté the onion and sunflower seeds in sunflower oil until onion is translucent and seeds are crisp. Combine noodles with sautéed onion and seeds.

Dissolve kuzu (or arrowroot) in water and heat, stirring until thick. Stir tofu, kuzu and seasonings into noodles. Place in oiled casserole dish. Bake for 25 minutes until firm. Top with No-Tomato Sauce and serve. *Serves 4.*

Broccoli soup   *5th Day Dinner*

2 quarts water
½ head broccoli
1 large onion
⅛ teaspoon salt
3 tablespoons olive oil
1 teaspoon tarragon

Bring water to a boil. Chop broccoli and onion into large pieces; add with salt and oil to water. Lower heat and simmer for 12–15 minutes. Separate vegetables from liquid and place in blender with a little water. Blend into a puree; return to soup pot, add tarragon and simmer 10 minutes longer on low heat. *Serves 4.*

No-tomato sauce on rice pasta   *5th Day Dinner*

Broiled Chicken Breast:
½ chicken breast with bone
1 clove garlic, peeled
Pinch of paprika
Pinch of pepper
Pinch of your favorite herb

Preheat broiler. Place chicken on greased broiler pan, rub with garlic, and sprinkle with paprika, pepper and herb of your choice. Broil for approximately 15 minutes (be sure to watch carefully). Dice into small pieces and set aside.

No-Tomato Sauce:
1 small beet, cubed
1 pound carrots, diced
2 onions, diced
1 bay leaf
1 tablespoon miso
2 cups water
½ teaspoon oregano
¼ teaspoon basil
½ teaspoon salt
2 cloves garlic
2 tablespoons arrowroot

Place beet, carrots and onion in pressure cooker. Add bay leaf. Dissolve miso in water and add to vegetables. Add 1 inch more of water, cover and pressure-cook for 15 minutes. Add seasonings and garlic. Remove vegetables and puree in blender, slowly adding cooking water as needed for texture. Put puree back into pressure cooker and heat uncovered. Add arrowroot, dissolved in ¼ cup water, to thicken. Simmer sauce 5–10 minutes, stirring occasionally. Add diced chicken to sauce.

Rice Pasta:
3 quarts water
½ teaspoon salt
12 ounces rice elbows

Bring water and salt to a boil. Cook noodles for 8–12 minutes and drain. Rinse well with cold water. Top with hot No-Tomato Sauce. *Serves 4.*

Chicken cubes with onions and vegetables   6th Day Lunch

1 tablespoon olive oil
6 ounces chicken, cut into small cubes
2 scallions, sliced small
1 onion, sliced in rounds
½ cup shredded cabbage
1 cup shredded kale
¼ teaspoon rosemary
¼ teaspoon ground ginger
¼ teaspoon oregano
Fresh parsley sprigs

In a skillet, heat oil and add chicken. Sauté until chicken is cooked all the way through. Cooking time depends on the tenderness of the meat and the size of the pieces; should be approximately 15 minutes. Remove from pan, saving meat juice.

Sauté scallions and onion in meat juice until transparent. Add shredded cabbage and kale. Add water if needed. Stir in seasonings. When vegetables begin to soften, stir in chicken and serve. Garnish with parsley sprigs. *Serves 2.*

String beans—boiled or steamed   6th Day Lunch

½ pound fresh string beans

Wash beans and snap off ends. Place in 2 quarts boiling water for approximately 5 minutes. Keep uncovered.

Or:

Bring 1 cup water to a boil and steam beans in stainless steel steamer basket until tender.

May be seasoned with a pinch of basil or tarragon. *Serves 4.*

Lima beans and quinoa   *6th Day Dinner*

1 cup cooked lima beans
⅔ cup cooked quinoa
¼ cup fresh chopped parsley
⅓ cup steamed chopped onions
1 tablespoon tarragon
¼ teaspoon salt

Combine all ingredients and mix well. May be served hot or cold. *Serves 2.*

Chinese tuna salad   *7th Day Lunch*

1 carrot
3–4 ounces water-packed tuna, drained
½ teaspoon basil
Pepper to taste
2–3 romaine lettuce leaves
Watercress
Radish slices

Wash carrot, peel if not organically grown and shred. Combine with tuna and seasoning and mix well. Serve on bed of lettuce garnished with watercress sprigs and radish slices.

Dressing:
1½ tablespoons olive oil
¼ cup chopped scallions
1 clove garlic, minced
1 cup chopped celery
½ onion, chopped
1 teaspoon Sesame Salt (see page 197)
1 teaspoon minced ginger

Heat oil and add scallions, garlic, celery and onion. Stir 5 minutes, adding water if needed. Sprinkle seasonings on top and fold into mixture. Serve over tuna salad. *Serves 2.*

Stuffed Cornish hen   *7th Day Dinner*

1 Cornish hen

Stuffing:
¼ cup diced celery
¼ red onion, chopped
⅛ teaspoon olive oil
1 cup partially cooked brown rice
1 handful raisins
⅓ teaspoon basil
⅛ teaspoon thyme
⅛ teaspoon sage

Sauté celery and onion in olive oil until slightly cooked. Combine with remaining ingredients, mix well and set aside.

Preheat oven to 350 degrees. Wash hen and remove excess fat. Stuff with rice mixture. Place in roasting pan, cover and roast for approximately 30 minutes. Uncover, baste with juice of bird and continue roasting for approximately 30 minutes more. The bird is cooked when golden brown and tender. *Serves 2.*

7

DIET TYPE 4

The Natural Raw Foods Diet

I was a teenager during the late great 1960s, when everyone around me seemed to be either turning vegetarian or at least heading in that direction. Some of the most dedicated converts to sprouts and raw greens had been confirmed cheeseburger lovers just a few years before. A renewed interest in the environment, however, prompted their searching for a more "enlightened," health-conscious way of eating. I was no exception. But while my generation may appear to have discovered the joys of whole, uncooked, unprocessed food (among other vegetarian virtues), this kind of diet has a long and venerable history.

Without getting into its ancient roots, we can date the "raw foods" tradition in this country to the Natural Hygiene Movement of the early 1830s. Dr. Herbert Shelton is credited with developing the first American food plan which relied mostly on fresh raw fruits and vegetables and set forth the principles of "conscious food combining." This involves eating foods in a certain sequence, from simple to more complex. The latest variation on this enduring theme is the much-talked-about *Fit for Life* diet, which promotes a number of basic Natural Hygiene principles. These include:

- avoiding or strictly limiting all animal fats, meat and dairy products;
- an emphasis on fresh, raw fruits and vegetables and their juices to obtain the benefits of natural enzymes;
- food combining and sequencing for digestive ease and efficiency;
- sprouting to enhance both the digestibility and nutritional content of legumes (peas and beans) and grains.

Not surprisingly, this kind of diet , with its focus on fresh, whole, high-fiber foods, either in their natural state or lightly cooked, is nutritious on many counts. The fluid-rich, low-fat meals are high in potassium and water-soluble vitamins (C and the B complex) and low in calories and sodium. This makes them excellent for those with a tendency to hypertension or high cholesterol. At Duke University, a closely supervised diet consisting largely of rice and fresh fruit markedly reduced blood pressure in patients with hypertension. Also noted was its beneficial effect on rheumatoid arthritis and gout.

In another study at the University Department of Medicine at Queen Elizabeth II Medical Center in Nedlands, Australia, patients with mild hypertension were placed on either a modified vegetarian diet (including low-fat dairy foods and eggs) or a typical omnivorous diet. The vegetarian regimen featured a higher ratio of polyunsaturated to saturated fat, an increase in fiber, calcium and magnesium, and a decrease in protein. Within six weeks, those on the vegetarian diet showed a significant reduction in systolic blood pressure. These readings returned to their elevated pretreatment levels when the subjects resumed their meat-based diets. The researchers concluded that the vegetarian diet should be recommended to people with mild hypertension.

For years, many European doctors have been claiming that since raw vegetables, fruits and juices are relatively simple foods, moderate in both protein and carbohydrates, they are less taxing to the system and can have a restorative, cleansing effect. I'll admit to having strong anecdotal evidence that they could be right. For example, I had a patient with chronic hepatitis who had been told by several physicians that he was inevitably headed for cirrhosis and eventual liver failure. As a first step I advised him to go on the Natural Raw Foods Diet and to get plenty of rest for several weeks. He purchased a Champion juicer and headed for Florida, where he subsisted on light foods, fruits and fresh vegetable juices. When he returned, he was fifteen pounds lighter and his formerly sallow skin had good color and luster. More important, his once-elevated liver enzymes registered normal—a sign that his disease was definitely under control.

The best vegetarian diets have been associated with lower rates of heart disease and cancer because they are sparing in saturated fats, cholesterol and animal proteins. They also feature eat-all-you-want portions of many foods. I describe the

COOL FOOD

When it's especially warm outdoors, eating smaller amounts of food throughout the day (five or six mini-meals) can keep you cooler than the traditional three square meals. This is because consuming a lot of food in one sitting promotes *thermogenesis,* a speeding up of the metabolism that raises body temperature slightly. Fluid-rich fruits and vegetables are ideal for summer snack-type eating and also help prevent hot-weather thirst and dehydration. Remember, *water in any form is a natural diuretic:* the more you ingest, the less fluid your tissues will retain.

Natural Raw Foods Diet as "lazy vegetarian," since, unlike Diet Type 1, it calls for little cooking or special preparation and is especially well suited for hot weather. While no one has proved the connection, many of us seem to make automatic adjustments in our diets during the summer, choosing foods that contain plenty of water, namely, fruits and vegetables. Our appetites probably diminish in such weather, too, because we require food for nourishment only, not warmth.

The premise of Diet Type 4 is that foods close to their natural state, as unadulterated and fresh as possible, are the best choices for growth, energy and the daily maintenance of all body systems. Overprocessing removes a tremendous amount of nutrients, including trace elements and fiber, and may expose us to harmful synthetic ingredients as well. Refined, low-fiber foods also encourage overeating, the argument goes, because they must be consumed in larger-than-usual amounts to satisfy a normal appetite.

Even among the "naturals," eating something whole is always preferable. Thus, whenever possible, it's better to have whole-grain breads and cereals than parts of them, like bran or wheat germ. For example, when integrated into the whole-wheat kernel, bran is an important nutritional element, but by itself or in excessive amounts it may be overly irritating.

Raw-foods advocates generally prefer the pectins in fruits and vegetables as sources of fiber. And nutritional science apparently favors them, too. Pectins are now considered a valuable group of fibers because they absorb bile salts, fats and cholesterol, thus increasing the rate at which these are removed from the body.

Cooking or heating destroys water-soluble vitamins. However, many foods are harder to digest in their uncooked state, so their nutrients are not always usable by the body. But when raw beans and grains are *sprouted,* they become far more digestible because enzymes known as trypsin inhibitors (which block the action of pancreatic enzymes) are destroyed in the process. Sprouting also increases vitamin content.

What do natural hygienists have against milk and other dairy products? The trouble, they say, is that milk is in a sense *unnatural,* for it is designed for cattle, not humans. These animals gain hundreds of pounds during the first few months of life and require a power-packed food, but the formula is far too rich for babies.* Generally, the smaller the species of animal, the more closely its milk resembles our own. Goat's milk, for example, is considered by some authorities to be nutritionally superior and more compatible with the human digestive tract.

While skim milk is less objectionable because it's free of saturated fat, some still consider its protein content more suited to calves than to people. Interestingly, studies have shown that casein, or milk protein, by itself can elevate blood cholesterol.

A great number of people are either allergic to milk or lactose intolerant. It's been argued, too, though not proved, that homogenization breaks down particles of saturated fat so finely that these may be small enough to penetrate the lining of blood vessels, where they can accumulate—possibly making inveterate milk drinkers more prone to heart disease. Strict natural hygienists don't like cheese or yogurt much, either, although they agree the latter is easier to digest than milk in any form.

While cow's milk may not be the perfect food, keep in mind that man is a uniquely *adaptable* animal, able to accommodate to a wide variety of foods and environments. If, however, you're convinced that milk isn't for you and you wish to cut down on dairy foods, how can you be sure to get enough calcium? Four cruciferous vegetables—turnip greens, broccoli, bok choy and collard greens—each supply more calcium per cup than does a half glass (4 ounces) of skim milk. (For other good sources of calcium among the "greens," consult the chart on page 236.)

Generally, the forbidden foods on Diet Type 4 include

---

* Newborns who are weaned on cow's milk formula are more susceptible to infections and milk-related allergies than those who are breast-fed.

salt, pepper, sugar (except the natural fructose in fruits), whole milk, cream, butter, egg yolks, ice cream, alcohol, soft drinks (including diet sodas), beef, pork and lamb. Vegetable oils and fats, strictly limited, should be "cold-pressed" or "extra virgin," that is, unadulterated by heat and chemical agents. Small amounts of fish, chicken or low-fat meats like veal or rabbit, along with part-skim cheeses and low-fat yogurt are permitted for those who will not be all-out vegetarians.

Vegetables are plentiful on Diet Type 4. Along with fruits, they provide nearly all the vitamin C available from food, and almost half the vitamin A. The latter is a must for healthy skin, a well-functioning gastrointestinal tract and reproductive system, and the proper development of bones and teeth. The darker green or deeper yellow the vegetable, the higher its concentration of vitamin A. Spinach is one of the best sources, providing the total RDA for adults in a single 2-ounce serving. Other good-to-excellent sources include broccoli, bok choy, asparagus, green beans, collard greens, fennel, lettuce and other salad greens, peas, Swiss chard, sweet potatoes, pumpkins and squash.

Vitamin C is required for maintaining teeth, capillaries, cell membranes and skin. It enhances the body's ability to absorb and use iron and also counteracts the effects of nitrosamines, potentially cancer-causing agents in the body. Cabbage, kohlrabi and brussels sprouts are rich in vitamin C, as are tomatoes, sweet green and red peppers and dark, leafy green vegetables.

All vegetables are good suppliers of iron, calcium, thiamine, niacin, potassium, magnesium, phosphorus and riboflavin as well as fiber and valuable trace elements. The cruciferous vegetables—broccoli, brussels sprouts, cabbage and cauliflower, among others—contain substances called indoles, which activate certain enzymes that help detoxify active carcinogens. The yellow vegetables, including squash, carrots, sweet potatoes, corn and pumpkins, along with parsley, watercress, romaine and spinach, are rich in beta-carotene, the raw material from which the body manufactures vitamin A. The amount of beta-carotene in leafy greens depends on the quantity of red, yellow and orange pigment; thus, the darkest in color are the richest nutritionally. As a group, carotene compounds, or carotenoids, are associated with protection from cancer, and many also suppress tumor formation.

Raw or cooked, vegetables are so filling and so low in calories, it's virtually impossible to overeat them. Whether you're a strictly-for-convenience cook or a painstaking gourmet, vegetables are delightfully versatile star performers in any number of dishes, including salads, soufflés, pastas, soups, stews and casseroles. And the cast of artful players seems to grow with every harvest; for example, jicama, white turnip, arugula, radicchio, daikon, black radish and Jerusalem artichokes are fast joining cucumbers, carrots and celery as salad-bowl staples.

Legumes and leafy greens are superior sources of folic acid, which is crucial to the formation of red blood cells and especially needed by expectant and nursing mothers. Raw produce is best, since cooking can destroy this B vitamin. If

PLANTS THAT PURIFY

A study at the Loma Linda University School of Medicine showed that plant fibers such as alfalfa meal help counteract the toxic effects of certain chemicals and food additives. Mice fed various harmful substances developed signs of serious illnesss while they were on a low-plant-fiber diet; however, the same dosages of these chemicals had no impact on animals fed a meal rich in plant fiber. Plant fiber is also associated with a significant decrease in blood cholesterol. This may partially explain why vegetarians consistently show a lower rate of heart disease than the average population.

mothers-to-be could be convinced to eat plenty of leafy greens throughout pregnancy and breast-feeding, the incidence of anemia would be dramatically reduced, according to a report entitled "Lettuce for Mothers" that appeared in the *British Medical Journal*.

Fruit is another mainstay on Diet Type 4. The firm, fragrant McIntosh, the plump, rosy-cheeked nectarine, the pink-to-perfection half grapefruit on the morning breakfast table have more than just eye and taste appeal: They also deliver a basketful of nutrients, including vitamin A, thiamine, niacin, vitamin B-6, folic acid, magnesium, iron, calcium and potassium, along with cholesterol-absorbing pectin. And they require little care in storage to preserve these benefits.

Even the sugar found in fruits is an advantage. Unlike refined white table sugar, it satisfies our natural craving for sweets without stimulating the pancreas to release too much insulin, which can cause sharp fluctuations in energy and mood.

Since Diet Type 4 is so rich in the fresh and natural, it's hard to imagine that some people may have problems with it. However, while it's far more desirable than a diet high in refined sugars and starches, it's still not the best possible choice for those with blood sugar disorders, because it has an unusually high level of fructose (fruit sugar). The latter raises blood glucose as well as triglyceride levels, although less dramatically than candies, cakes, cookies, honey and other refined sweets. Those with recurring yeast infections (candidiasis) should watch their fruit-sugar intake as well. Moreover, raw foods are not always easy to digest, which may discourage older people or those with a tendency to weak digestion. Some eaters may not find the salad emphasis hearty or satisfying enough to curb their hunger during colder months. The diet is hard to travel with, too, and may be inconvenient if you're largely dependent on hotel and restaurant meals. It works best for those who can shop for fresh fruits and vegetables frequently.

Popular versions of Diet Type 4 have stressed the careful

timing and arranging of foods in a certain order—a ritual that's inconvenient at best and potentially unhealthful, even risky, at worst. The practice is based on the (long-discredited) belief that sequential eating and food combining can help conserve the energy used by the body for the digestion and absorption of foods, while maximizing the energy needed for healing and repair. Proponents of this principle insist that the simplest foods should be eaten first, followed by the more complex ones: For instance, a raw, unpeeled fruit or a leafy green salad would precede a dish of nuts or low-fat cheese. Another cardinal rule is that a carbohydrate and a protein should never be eaten in the same meal: A turkey sandwich, for example, would be prohibited. Those who violate this dietary caveat are warned that the mixture of these foods will stagnate and ferment in the stomach—and encourage weight gain—since the body secretes only one digestive enzyme at a time and can't handle both substances. Nonsense! We are exquisitely capable of handling many types of diets and every conceivable combination of natural food. (Of course, some of today's synthetic foods certainly give our digestive apparatus a run for its money!)

A variety of digestive enzymes are released automatically whenever food enters the stomach. Each enzyme performs a multiplicity of functions and does not have to hold center stage to do its work. Thus, proteins, carbohydrates and fats can be worked on simultaneously; none of them has to wait in the wings. This means you can eat foods in whatever order or combinations you want—it makes no difference to your stomach or state of health, nor will it add a single extra ounce of weight. In fact, some highly nutritious foods, such as bread, legumes, milk and nuts, are a natural blend of proteins and carbohydrates.

While the Natural Hygiene diet is clearly beneficial, its advocates have often cloaked it in pseudoscience. Sometimes the myth has bordered on the outright harmful. For example, one recently popularized diet calls for eating only fruit until noon, a rule that can pose serious problems for diabetics, hypoglycemics, the elderly, and pregnant or lactating women. Other people following this fruit-only formula may simply feel fatigued, washed out, unable to perform at their best—and all because of folklore!

The notion that raw vegetables, fruits and juices are sources of essential "enzymes" that the body requires is likewise unfounded. These enzymes are peculiar to plants and have little importance inside our bodies. It's not true that grapefruit enzymes can digest away fat, as some diet books have claimed. In fact, nearly all plant enzymes are digested in their entirety by the time they reach the small intestine, where their molecules are absorbed into the bloodstream along with amino acids, sugars, minerals, vitamins and fats.

What's more, some people go overboard in the hope of "detoxifying" their bodies. I have seen several patients who courted malnutrition by staying on strict "cleansing" regimens of only salad and fruit. Some of them experienced lean-muscle loss, dry skin, thinning hair and fatigue. Others

STOMACH-LOVING VEGGIES

A University of Southampton study published in the *British Medical Journal** reveals that green vegetables, rich in a type of fiber that is kindly to intestinal bacteria, may discourage appendicitis. Researchers studying population groups in both England and Wales showed that a steady diet of cabbage, cauliflower, peas, beans and brussels sprouts offered the greatest protection against this painful malady. Interestingly, diets high in cereal fiber did not prevent the condition, while frequent meals of potatoes were associated with an increased risk.

* April 5, 1986, as reported in *HealthFacts*, a newsletter of the Center for Medical Consumers in New York City.

THE SUBJECT IS LEAFY GREENS

All are first-rate sources of vitamins A and C and folic acid (an anti-anemia B vitamin); they're also good suppliers of vitamins D, B-6, riboflavin, thiamine, niacin, iron, calcium and other minerals, are low in calories and are fine sources of fiber as well as good-quality protein.

A slight catch? You might have heard that some leafy greens, such as spinach, contain oxalates or oxalic acid, which binds some of their calcium and iron and makes them unavailable to the body. The presence of oxalates may also decrease the availability of these minerals from other foods eaten at the same meal. However, according to the American Medical Association's Department of Foods and Nutrition, it is unlikely many people eat spinach (and other oxalate-containing vegetables, such as dandelion, parsley and beet greens) in the amounts necessary to interfere with calcium and iron absorption.

For a fresh slaw, chop raw cabbage, carrots, celery (including the leaves), any greens, cucumbers and red and green peppers. Marinate in vinegar diluted with water to taste. Season with sea salt, pepper, paprika or other condiments. Refrigerate; can be used with any fish, poultry or cheese.

showed signs of anemia, as well as vitamin and protein deficiencies. The sicker they become, the more convinced they are that further dietary restrictions are necessary to drive out residual "toxins." One patient rallied with a healthful 20 pound weight gain in two weeks just by adding whole grains and legumes at my urging.

Is there *any* merit to food combining? To those few patients of mine who have complained of severe flatulence and bloating or poor digestion, I have suggested one Natural Hygiene principle that apparently helps: eating fruits or drinking fruit juices at least a half hour before and two hours after a meal. For those with normal digestion, however, this guideline is unnecessary. As a weight-loss strategy, food combining can be useful because it imposes some rules and discipline on the dieter, forcing him or her to plan meals with care and discouraging compulsive, mindless eating.

Because of their restrictions on dairy products, meat and fish, popular forms of this diet category may be low in calcium, iron and vitamin B-12. Too many raw vegetables and fruits may pose a drawback for people with higher-than-average protein requirements, such as growing children and teenagers, highly athletic men and women, and pregnant and/or lactating women, as well as the elderly, who may not be so scrupulous about eating a balanced diet or who may simply have trouble chewing certain foods. The Diet Type 4 menu plan draws on the best features of other natural-foods diets and corrects the imbalances associated with the well-known versions of this basically nutritious food regimen. It has the highest water content of the diets in this book, making it naturally satisfying, and it is also the least calorie-dense. Included are fruits that are relatively low in sugar, seasonal produce for maximum nutritional benefit, just enough seafood and olive oil to control triglycerides, and sprouted legumes, low-fat dairy products, soy foods and some grains for adequate protein.

THE PICK OF THE RAW FOODS DIET

Since this diet focuses on fruits and vegetables, these guidelines are aimed at helping you have the best of both, from picking to preparation.*

* Some of the information in this section, along with the suggestions on picking fresh vegetables and fruits, is derived in part from the excellent consumer publications available from the United Fresh Fruit and Vegetable Association, North Washington at Madison, Alexandria, VA 22314, and the Grand Union Company, 333 North Bedford Rd., Mt. Kisco, NY.

■ It doesn't take special know-how to judge the freshness of produce or its readiness for eating. Appearances *aren't* deceiving: Vegetables and fruits that look most appealing are likely to be the most nutritious and flavorful. In general, look for taut, unbroken skins or flesh, with even shapes, vibrant colors and no evidence of shriveling, bruising, cracking, soft spots, rotting or rusting. Leaf and flower clusters should be tightly furled and not yellowed, stem ends moist and free of browning. Fresh herbs and leafy greens should be bright and lively looking, with no signs of wilting or discoloration.

■ If possible, buy fresh vegetables and fruits from greengrocers and farmers' markets or from supermarkets that get daily deliveries, even though they may be a bit more expensive. They're not only tastier but are also more likely to be free of produce-ripening chemicals.

■ To remove oil-based sprays and resins, wash fruits and vegetables in a little soapy water, then rinse thoroughly.

Eat the skins of vegetables and fruits whenever possible, since they contain a large proportion of the nutrients. A vegetable brush will wash away dirt and surface residues. Potatoes lose 25 percent of their vitamin C when you peel the skin; removing the pith or white part of the skin around an orange eliminates much of its vitamin C. Leaving on the skin and pith of fruits also ensures that you'll be getting beneficial pectin.

■ Eat plenty of greens. Today you have more choices than ever and greengrocers abound as never before. Watercress, spinach, dandelion, mustard and collard greens, escarole, arugula, romaine, kale and Chinese cabbage are all superior to the paler iceberg lettuce. Remember, the darker green the vegetable, the more nutrients, especially vitamins A and C, it contains.

■ Avoid buying packages of prechopped vegetables for soups, stews and sandwiches, since they may have already lost too many valuable nutrients in the cutting process.

■ If you buy prepared vegetables or fruits, pick the plain quick-frozen kind, without added sugar, sauce or syrups.

■ Never overcook vegetables. Steam or boil them in a small

amount of water until they are crisp to tender. Or stir- or panfry them in a little extra-virgin olive oil with fresh garlic and your favorite herbs. Save leftover juices, rich in water-soluble nutrients, for use as a base in soups and stews. Or add extra flavor to vegetables by braising them—adding a small amount of tomato sauce or stock, covering the pan and allowing them to steam in flavorful liquid. Cook fleshy vegetables such as squash and broccoli until crisply tender, then puree and season. The result will seem richer than it actually is and can be served as a side dish or used as the base for a soup or sauce.

▪ Growing bean sprouts at home is a way of obtaining truly fresh, live food even in midwinter! Place any kind of beans in a wide-mouthed jar and soak them with water. Cover the jar with nylon mesh or cheesecloth and discard the water the next morning. Rinse and drain the beans twice daily and store in a warm, dark place for two to four days. Or use a commercial sprouter, available in kitchen-supply and some health-food stores.

▪ For maximum nutritional value, keep greens cold, moist and crisp. Sprinkle, don't soak, them with ice water and wrap in a damp cloth in the refrigerator to help preserve their vitamin C. Lightly wash—don't discard—the dark outer leaves of lettuce and other greens since these contain up to fifty times more vitamin A than the inner white ones, as well as considerably more vitamin C and calcium. Likewise, don't throw away broccoli leaves: Very tasty and nutritious, they have twenty times more vitamin A than the stalk and several times as much as the florets. Steam them for about fifteen minutes with the florets.

▪ For most vegetables, careful cold storage is essential. Cold, but not freezing, temperatures slow the action of internal enzymes that may cause flesh, stems, bulbs, leaves or roots to soften or lose color. They also retard evaporation of the vegetables' natural moisture through the skin.

▪ Broccoli, lima beans, squash, sweet corn, asparagus and spinach lose moisture easily and should be refrigerated immediately.

■ Beets, turnips and carrots should be stored without their tops attached, since they give up moisture (and nutrients) through these natural "pipelines." However, leave the stem scar on a tomato, if possible, so it can hold its moisture longer.

■ Don't refrigerate potatoes and hard-rind squash; instead, store in a cool, dry place. Keep unripe tomatoes at room temperature until they're ripe, then either eat immediately or refrigerate.

■ The color of greens is lost when chlorophyll breaks down due to heat and acid; the shorter the cooking time, the less greenness is lost. To preserve color and nutrients, boil quickly in a small amount of water (just enough to avoid scorching), keeping the lid off the pot during the first few minutes to allow the volatile acids to escape. Or use a steamer or pressure cooker. Don't add baking soda to retain the green color; it destroys vitamin C and the B complex vitamins.

■ Don't discard cauliflower or radish leaves if these are in good condition; both are surprisingly high in protein.

■ Fibrous parts of leaves such as the stems and ribs are less palatable and have fewer nutrients than the thin part. The leaves of collard greens, for example, are not only more tender than the midrib, but have also been found to contain thirty times as much vitamin A.

■ Use a sharp knife to cut vegetables: A dull utensil bruises them and thus hastens the loss of valuable nutrients.

■ Don't worry about eating fresh citrus fruit (or any other kind) on an empty stomach, despite the myths about acid content. The natural hydrochloric acid in your stomach is far more acidic than anything you could eat, including even straight lime or lemon juice.

■ If you cannot use fresh vegetables while they're in top condition, cook them lightly (by steaming, stir-frying or blanching) to extend their shelf life, then use them in salads, soups, stuffings or sauces.

■ Avoid cooking with copper pots and pans, since these accelerate the loss of vitamin C.

Raw vs. Cooked

While raw produce does provide nutrients in their unadulterated state, light cooking can make some foods more digestible and allow their minerals to be better absorbed. Kale is a good example of a nutritionally valuable plant that is scarcely palatable when raw, but which is easily assimilated after steaming or pressure-cooking. Sprouting raw beans and seeds makes them easier to digest and also enhances their vitamin content.

■ Some of the iron in plants is bound up in such a way as to be poorly absorbed compared with the iron from animal sources. Eating foods rich in vitamin C at the same meal (namely, fruits and vegetables) will help enhance iron absorption.

Is Organic Produce Better?

The answer is yes and no. On the one hand, organic fruits and vegetables sold in health-food stores and greengrocers' markets are relatively free of pesticides, a plus for safe eating. However, large supermarket chains have a more efficient means of distributing their foods, delivering them over larger distances in a shorter time. Thus, regular produce may be fresher and livelier, less bruised and wilted and possibly higher in nutrients because of its better condition. The best option—growing your own—is only open to some.

▪ Vitamin B-12 is found in all food of animal origin, but not in vegetables or fruits. If you're a strict vegetarian, brewer's yeast, textured vegetable protein, breakfast cereals, soybean tempeh or natto and kombu and wakame (Japanese seaweeds) will supply B-12.

▪ Getting enough vitamin D, a fat-soluble vitamin not found in vegetables or fruits, is a concern primarily for the housebound and elderly, growing children and expectant mothers, who should drink vitamin D–fortified milk or take supplements. If you're spending a reasonable amount of time outdoors, your body is probably synthesizing enough. If you're at risk, though, for insurance take a daily multivitamin supplement containing 400 IUs of vitamin D.

VEGETABLES: HOW TO PICK THE FRESHEST

ARTICHOKES: Choose compact, heavy, plump globes with large, tightly clinging leaf scales of olive green color. (Size makes little difference.) When petals are open and spreading, they're overmature and tough.

ASPARAGUS: Spears should be fresh, firm and slender, with compact, closed tips. Select spears with a large amount of green.

BEANS, SNAP: Pods should be firm, crisp and slender with good green color. Avoid beans with scars.

BROCCOLI: Look for compact bud clusters. Color varies from dark green to sage green to purplish green, depending on the variety. Yellow and wilted leaves indicate aging.

BRUSSELS SPROUTS: These should be firm, compact and with bright leaves. Avoid wilted or yellow leaves.

CABBAGE: Heads should be reasonably solid and

(Continued)

(Continued)

heavy in relation to size, with green hard outer leaves (except, of course, red cabbage). Leaves separating at the base may indicate age or poor storage. A good buy during winter, when other vegetables are generally higher-priced.

CARROTS: Look for firm, well-shaped roots with a good orange color. Remove the tops to maintain moisture, since water evaporates through these natural outlets. Fresh market carrots are usually smaller, more tender and brighter than those harvested for storage. (The latter are okay for shredding and cooking.)

CAULIFLOWER: White or creamy-white firm, compact clusters indicate good quality. Size of head is unimportant.

CELERY: Choose fresh, crisp, smooth stalks that are thick and solid (rough ones may be harder to chew); light green stalks are tastiest. To preserve freshness and crispness, cut into individual stalks and immerse in a container of water in the refrigerator.

CORN, SWEET: Buy in season, locally. Select only corn that is cold to the touch. (The sugar in unrefrigerated picked corn turns to starch in a few hours, so that it's no longer sweet-tasting. It also loses vitamin C after a few days.) Buy it on the day you plan to eat it. If it must be kept, leave it in the husk and wrap in plastic before refrigerating it. Husks should be green, not dry or yellowish.

CUCUMBERS: Look for medium sizes with good green color. Avoid very large, puffy ones or any having a yellow color. To retain vitamin C, don't slice until ready to eat.

EGGPLANT: Should be firm and heavy for their size, with dark purple to purple black skin. Wrinkling or softness indicates a bitter or lackluster flavor as well

(Continued)

(Continued)

as nutrition loss. Short cooking time will help conserve vitamin C and folic acid.

ENDIVE/ESCAROLE/CHICORY: Should be fresh, clean, crisp and cold. Avoid dry, yellowing or wilted leaves, or those showing reddish discoloration of the hearts.

GREENS (Collard, Turnip, Dandelion, Mustard, Beet, Kale): Choose fresh young and crisp green leaves. Avoid any with coarse stems or wilted, yellowing leaves. Greens of all kinds contain a good deal of vitamin C, folic acid and vitamin A, as well as minerals. Particularly to preserve the vitamin C, they need to be refrigerated promptly and at high humidity until they are cooked or eaten. The thin part of the leaves may contain twenty times as much vitamin A, many times more vitamin C and two to four times more iron than the midribs, which are more fibrous and less edible.

KOHLRABI: The stem should be medium-sized and firm, with green, crisp tops.

LEEKS: Choose small or medium leeks and well-blanched bunches for the most tender eating. Refrigerate in a plastic bag and use within three to five days.

LETTUCE (iceberg): Justly maligned because of its low nutritional content, this is basically "crunch" and little else.

LETTUCE (other): Select clean, fresh and tender heads. When chopped, any kind of lettuce loses ascorbic and folic acid much faster than when leaves are whole, so don't shred far in advance of use. The greener the leaves, the more vitamins A and C and other nutrients they contain. Discard only the damaged outer ones and refrigerate to retain nutritional value.

(Continued)

(Continued)

MUSHROOMS: May be white, tan or cream-colored. Refrigerate and cover with a damp paper towel to help retain moisture. Avoid storing in plastic bags, since this hampers air circulation. Mushrooms do not store well, so it is best to use them promptly. They lose few nutrients if cooked briefly in a small amount of water.

OKRA: Pods should be young and tender, preferably 2 to 4 inches long. Avoid dull, dry or shriveled pods.

ONIONS (yellow, white, red, Bermuda): Choose bulbs that are clean and firm. The skins should be dry, smooth and crackly. Avoid onions with wet, soggy necks or soft, spongy bulbs, which are signs of decay. Keep at slightly cool temperature in a well-ventilated area. Onions may be refrigerated; above all, keep them dry. They can be stored three to four weeks.

ONIONS (green): Select young and tender bunches with fresh green tops. Keep refrigerated in a plastic bag and use as soon as possible.

PEPPERS: Should be fresh, firm and thick-fleshed, with bright green coloring that may be tinged with red. Immature peppers are usually soft and dull-looking. Green peppers are high in vitamin C, and mature red peppers are very high in both C and A.

POTATOES: Choose firm, clean and relatively smooth ones free of cuts or bruises. Avoid green-colored potatoes and those with buds or sprouts. Never refrigerate, but keep in a cool, well-ventilated area. Keep away from light (which can cause greening) and moisture. Potatoes are an important source of vitamin C, second only to citrus fruits. *Sweet potatoes* are an excellent source of beta-carotene (a forerunner of vitamin A) and vitamin C. They should not be refrigerated, because they develop internal discoloration and decay.

(Continued)

(Continued)

RADISHES: All sizes and shapes should be fresh, smooth and well-formed, with few cuts, pits or black spots. Avoid spongy radishes.

SPINACH: Leaves should be clean and fresh, dark green in color. Avoid large yellow leaves and those that are wilted or discolored in any way.

SQUASH *(soft-skinned, or summer):* Should be fresh, heavy for its size and tender. Choose small to medium sizes. Refrigerate and use as soon as possible.

SQUASH (hard-shelled, or winter): Avoid any with soft areas. Hubbards can be stored six months or longer; acorn squash, three to six months. Keep in a dry, well-ventilated area at room temperature. Don't refrigerate.

STRING BEANS: Small, smooth ones are best; bumps denote toughness.

TOMATOES: Choose firm, smooth, unbruised and plump-looking tomatoes with good color and stems attached. Most tomatoes require further ripening at home. Place away from direct sunlight. Putting tomatoes in a bag hastens ripening. Don't refrigerate until fully red-ripe, then use within a few days. *Note:* Tomatoes grown outdoors may have twice as much vitamin C as those grown in winter greenhouses.

CALORIES AND SODIUM

The advantage of a diet high in fresh vegetables is their low calorie content, especially when compared to their nutrient levels. This makes them nutritionally dense, with great food value packed into each calorie. Even the starchier vegetables, like potatoes, are relatively low in calories; a medium-

---

WHAT'S UP, DOC?

The fiber content of just two medium carrots a day can help keep cholesterol under control. Try them raw, baked, steamed or sautéed, toss them in salads or grate them with apples, cabbage and raisins. Other cholesterol-reducing veggies and fruits are broccoli, beans, peas, onions, apples, oranges and grapefruit.

---

sized baking potato contains only about 110. Potatoes become fattening only if prepared or served with the fat in butter, oil, cream, sour cream or cheese. Similarly, watch out for tossed salads with thick, creamy or oil-based dressings, along with extras like croutons, bacon bits or cheese; all these can result in up to 800 additional calories!

Most vegetables are also low in sodium. Take advantage of this natural plus by seasoning them with fresh herbs and garlic, lemon or lime juice, ginger, hot peppers, onions or vinegar—no salt necessary! Avoid eating these sodium-rich vegetables too often if you must stick to a very stringent low-sodium diet: artichokes, beets, kale, spinach, Swiss chard, turnips and celery.

HIGH-CALCIUM VEGETABLES

Turnip greens, broccoli, bok choy and collard greens supply more calcium per cup than does a 4-ounce glass of milk. For a more complete list, see chart on page 236.

FRUITS: HOW TO PICK THE FRESHEST

Texture and aroma are prime considerations when selecting fruit. Also, keep your eye on the calendar: Many varieties will be at their best in both flavor and nutrition during their own peak season.

- Select evenly shaped fruit; misshapen produce is usually inferior in taste and texture.
- Look for fruit that has a good color and is free of stains, bruises, blemishes or soft spots; such damage accelerates decay and loss of nutrients. Brown speckling, called "russeting," is normal in some fruits, such as apples, bananas, pears, necatrines and citrus fruits, and often indicates a sweeter taste.
- Store unripe fruits at room temperature until they are ripe, then either eat or refrigerate them immediately.
- Don't wash any fruit until you're ready to use it, since the moisture promotes decay; this is especially true of soft-skinned fruit like cherries, grapes and plums.
- When fruits like apples, bananas, peaches and pears are cut, put orange or lemon juice on them to keep them from turning brown. The ascorbic acid in citrus acts as a natural food preservative.

APPLES: Look for firm, smooth and unwrinkled skin and keep cold to minimize loss of vitamin C.
AVOCADOS: These should be firm and hard, with no pitting or bruises on the skin. Depending on the variety, the skin may be smooth and glossy green, mottled with brown, or corrugated and nearly black. Avocados are ripe when they yield slightly to the touch. Under-

(Continued)

(Continued)

ripe avocados can be ripened at room temperature at home.

BANANAS: Fruit should be plump and firm, the skin unbroken and without bruises. Underripe bananas will mature perfectly at room temperature, so you may prefer to buy them on the green side. Bananas that become overripe can be mashed for use in baking breads, muffins and cakes.

BERRIES: Plump, full-colored berries will have the best flavor. Check the bottoms of the containers or baskets for signs of leaking or staining, and avoid bruised, shriveled or moldy fruit. Sort berries to remove any soft ones as soon as you get them home, but do not rinse until ready to use. Hull strawberries after washing.

Strawberries, raspberries, blackberries, boysenberries, loganberries, gooseberries and currants should be used within a day of purchase; blueberries will last a couple of days.

CHERRIES: Select ones that are firm, glossy and deep red to blackish in color. They should be free of soft or sticky spots; stems should be green, pliable and fresh-looking.

CITRUS FRUITS: All are ripe when picked; green skin does not indicate immaturity. Citrus fruits should be firm, thin-skinned and glossy; one that feels heavy for its size will have more juice. When whole, citrus fruits keep their vitamin C well without refrigeration for one or two weeks; with refrigeration, they can retain vitamin C for up to twelve weeks.

FIGS: These should be fairly soft, with no broken skin, and should have a pleasant fragrance, with no sour or fermented smell.

GRAPES: Firm, plump grapes without soft spots,

(Continued)

(Continued)

wrinkles or blemishes are best. They should be attached securely to pliable stems. Green grapes that have a slight amber tint will be sweeter. Gently shake a bunch; few will drop off if they're fresh.

KIWIS: These are ripe when soft but not mushy. They can mature at room temperature at home. Avoid kiwis with wrinkled skin.

MANGOES: Mangoes ripen well at room temperature, becoming quite soft, with large areas of pinkish, red and yellow on the skin. Avoid fruits with mushy spots, black pitting or gray discolorations. A ripe mango has a rich perfume, but a pungent or sour aroma means it is overripe.

MELONS: Ripe melons will yield slightly to pressure, especially at the ends, and have a sweet fragrance. Select melons that are uniform in shape. Depending on the variety, the color should be light green to yellow or cream. Except for watermelons, which should be lighter on the bottom, the color should be uniform.

Cantaloupes and Persian melons have a pattern of fine netting covering the skin, which should be pale and creamy in cantaloupes and greenish in Persian melons. Crenshaw and honeydew melons should be velvety-looking, the crenshaw light green to bright yellow and the honeydew a pale, creamy color. Honeydews are the only melons that continue to ripen after they have been picked. Other varieties may become juicier if left at room temperature for a day or two, but will not ripen further.

Note: Watermelon is not just water and sugar, but has a surprising amount of nutrients. An average-sized wedge provides half the recommended daily allowance for vitamin A and two-thirds of the vitamin C, as

(Continued)

(Continued)

well as a fifth of the iron recommended for a male adult. Keep it cold and use it soon. Look for juicy, fine-textured red flesh that is wet, not mealy, and studded with jet-black seeds.

PAPAYAS: Fruit should be at least half yellow when bought. Allow it to ripen at room temperature and make sure it turns completely yellow before using.

PEARS: The skin color of a ripe pear can vary from green to brown to red to gold, depending on the variety. Select pears that are firm but yield slightly to the touch at the stem end.

PINEAPPLES: As with many other fruits, once a pineapple is picked it will not ripen further. Look for one with a full crown of fresh green leaves. If one of the leaves is easily removed, the fruit is ready to eat. Also, smell the bottom: A pineappley fragrance is a sign of mature fruit. Color does not necessarily indicate ripeness—the large hawaiian "Sugar Loaf" variety can be green when fully ripe. Small pineapples should be more pinkish-gold than green. Avoid any with soft bottoms, bruises or oozing.

STONE FRUITS (Apricots, Nectarines, Peaches, Plums): Plump, sound fruit, free of bruises or soft spots, that yields slightly to the touch will be ready to eat. Avoid fruit that is greenish (except for Kelsey-Wicksom plums) and very hard, because it probably will not ripen properly. A red blush on peaches and nectarines does not denote ripeness.

HIGH-CALCIUM VEGETABLES

Vegetable	Milligrams of Calcium per 100 grams (3½ ounces)	Other Good Nondairy Sources	Milligrams of Calcium per 100 Grams (3 ½ ounces)
Kelp	1,093	Carob Flour	352
Dulse	296	Barbados	
Collard Greens	250	Molasses	245
Turnip Greens	246	Almonds	234
Parsley	203	Brewer's Yeast	210
Dandelion		Corn Tortillas	
Greens	187	(lime added)	200
Watercress	151	Brazil Nuts	186
Beet Greens	119	Tofu	128
Ripe Olives	106	Dried Figs	126
Broccoli	103	Sunflower Seeds	120
Romaine Lettuce	68	Wheat Bran	119
Rutabaga	66	Buckwheat, raw	114
Green Snap		Sesame Seeds,	
Beans	56	hulled	110
Globe Artichokes	51	English Walnuts	99
Green Cabbage	49	Pecans	73
Soybean Sprouts	48	Wheat Germ	72
Celery	39	Peanuts	69
Carrots	37	Miso	68
Summer Squash	28	Dried Apricots	67
Onion	27	Raisins	62
Fresh Green		Black Currants	60
Peas	26	Dates	59
Cauliflower	25	Dried Prunes	51
Asparagus	22	Pumpkin &	
		Squash Seeds	51
		Cooked Soy	
		Beans	50

QUICK FRUIT IDEAS

At breakfast, use fruit in cereal, muffin mixes or pancakes.

At lunch, add cut-up apples, pears or oranges to salad greens.

At dinner, add apple pieces or fresh pineapple slices to cole slaw.

Between meals, choose fruits in place of other foods high in sugar, fat and salt. Spread one or two teaspoons of freshly made unsalted peanut butter on apple slices for a satisfying protein/fiber snack.

GREEN WATER: THE NATURAL PURIFIER

Fat cells often act as a depot for toxic residues. As they break down during dieting, their contents are released and the temporary results can be headaches, fatigue and joint pain. Drinking "green water," a natural source of fresh chlorophyll and vitamins, is a beneficial way to flush these toxins out of the body. To prepare, combine one-half cup of vegetable greens such as celery, romaine lettuce, parsley, mint, sprouts and/or watercress with one and a half cups of distilled water in a blender for one minute. Then pour the mixture through a strainer and stir slowly.

Green water is best when freshly prepared, but will keep up to eight hours in the refrigerator. Use it as a refreshing pick-me-up on an empty stomach. (Avoid using it after food, as it may cause intestinal rumbling or even diarrhea.) It alleviates hunger pangs and fatigue, and is an excellent alternative to stimulants and sweets.

———————————— ▪ ————————————

SAMPLE MENUS

Recipes are provided for all dishes marked with an asterisk (*). To find recipes that appear in other sections, consult the Index at the back of this book.

Beverages for all meals: herbal tea, decaffeinated coffee, instant grain coffee (e.g., Caffix), skim milk, soy milk, seltzer, plain or sparkling mineral water, fresh vegetable juices or filtered tap water.

DAY 1:

Breakfast

⅔ cup crispy brown rice cereal with ⅓ to ⅔ cup Nut Milk*

Lunch

Zesty Broccoli-Spinach Salad*

½ cup steamed brown rice with chopped dill and sesame seeds

Dinner

½ cup Pasta Vegetable Medley*

Broccoli with Lemon Sauce* *or* Roasted Red Peppers*

Escarole and endive salad with lemon, fresh minced garlic and olive oil

Snack

½ papaya with fresh blueberries *or* ½ any fresh fruit in season

DAY 2:

Breakfast

8 ounces Fresh Fruit Shake*

Lunch

Raw Vegetable Salad with Peanut Sauce*

½ cup Guacamole Spread* on sprouted-wheat bread

Dinner

1 serving Broccoli-Cashew Tostada*

Assorted raw vegetables (cauliflower, bell peppers, carrots, zucchini, cherry tomatoes, broccoli, asparagus, celery, scallions) with 1 ounce crumbled feta or goat cheese, chopped fresh parsley, and apple cider, tarragon or balsamic vinegar

Snack

1 cup Green Water (see page 237)

DAY 3:

Breakfast

1 slice Sprouted-Wheat and Carrot Bread* with

1 tablespoon pureed fresh fruit *or* 1 tablespoon apple butter

Lunch

Four-Sprout Salad*

1 serving Spicy Onion-Mushroom Spread* with celery sticks

Dinner

1 serving South American Seviche*

Wonderful Waldorf Salad*

Snack

1½ tablespoons sliced almonds and raw sunflower seeds

DAY 4:

Breakfast

Tropical Fruit Cup with Creamy Topping*

2 rice cakes with 2 teaspoons cashew nut butter

Lunch

Avocado Salad*

Dinner

Baked Nut Loaf*

Colorful Coleslaw with Vinegar-Sesame Dressing*

Mixed Sprouts and Tofu*

Snack

Tropical "Smoothie"* drink *or* instant carrot juice (available at health-food stores)

DAY 5:

Breakfast

⅔ cup Muesli (see page 97) with ½ cup soy milk

Lunch

Salmon Spinach Salad*

Dinner

Light Tabouli Salad* *or* Great Gazpacho*

Tossed Delight Salad*

Snack

1 cup Green Water (see page 237)

DAY 6:

Breakfast

¼ cup almonds, walnuts and cashews

½ cup sliced fresh cantaloupe

Lunch

1 cup chickpea and onion salad (green-leaf lettuce, sliced tomatoes, chopped celery and onions with cooked or canned chickpeas)

1 serving Baba Ghanoush* on romaine leaves

Dinner

½ cup Cold Pasta Salad* *or* Special Herbed Potato Salad*

Steamed fresh vegetable mélange with garlic, lemon juice, cayenne and paprika

Snack

1 apple and 6 almonds

DAY 7:

Breakfast

½ banana, sliced lengthwise, sprinkled with 1 table-spoon crushed peanuts

Lunch

Cold Zucchini Salad*

1 slice whole-wheat bread

Dinner

Sesame Bluefish Stuffed Tomatoes*

Vegetables Marinade*

Snack

6 walnuts

---■---

FIVE EASY PIECES

Satisfying, nutritious, portable lunch/dinner alternatives that you can prepare with a minimum of fuss and effort. Each makes 1 individual portion.

1. Watercress salad
Dress together the following ingredients:
¾ cup watercress
1 tablespoon chopped walnuts
¼ cup sliced bamboo shoots
¼ cup mung bean sprouts
1 teaspoon low-sodium soy sauce
½ teaspoon dark sesame oil

2. *Avocado tostada*

   Whole-corn tostada shells are available from health-food stores. Stuff shells with mashed avocado, tomato, alfalfa sprouts, shredded romaine lettuce and grated carrots; add hot chili sauce.

3. *Apple spread*

   Peel ½ Red Delicious apple, mash thoroughly. Mix with 1 teaspoon unsweetened grated coconut, 1 teaspoon toasted sesame seeds and 1 teaspoon grape juice. Serve on Kavli flatbread or whole-wheat matzo.

4. *Sprout bread italiano*

   Top slices of sprouted whole-grain bread with mixture of ½ finely chopped tomato, ¼ finely chopped onion, 2–3 finely minced raw mushrooms, ½ teaspoon extra-virgin olive oil and a pinch of garlic powder, basil and oregano.

5. *Endive salad*

   Mix together ¾ cup chopped endive, ¼ cup grated carrots, 1 dozen raisins, 3 chopped whole pecans and 1 tablespoon eggless mayonnaise (available at health-food stores).

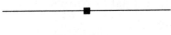

RECIPES

Nut milk	1st Day Breakfast

¼ cup cashews
¼ cup almonds
1½ cups spring water

Place cashews, almonds and 1 cup water in blender. Blend at medium-high speed, stopping occasionally to allow nuts to sink to the bottom. Slowly add remaining water and continue blending until mixture is creamy. Use ⅓–⅔ cup Nut Milk for each serving of cereal. *Yield: 2 cups*

Zesty broccoli-spinach salad   1st Day Lunch

2 cups spinach
8 ounces tofu cake, cubed
½ medium red onion, sliced
⅔ cup chopped, blanched broccoli florets
2 tablespoons olive oil
1 teaspoon tarragon
½ teaspoon salt
3 red radishes, thinly sliced
Juice of 1 lemon

Wash spinach carefully, remove stems and tear into large pieces. Sauté tofu, onion and broccoli in olive oil with tarragon and salt for 5–8 minutes, then combine with spinach and radishes. Add lemon juice and toss. Serve with brown rice. *Serves 4.*

Pasta vegetable medley   1st Day Dinner

8 ounces whole-grain pasta elbows, cooked
½ cup cut cauliflower
¼ cup sliced celery
2 scallions, chopped
1 tomato, diced
1 tablespoon olive oil
2 teaspoons natural soy (shoyu) sauce
¼ teaspoon grated ginger
¼ teaspoon oregano
Lemon juice

Mix ingredients well and sprinkle with a little lemon juice. *Serves 4.*

Broccoli with lemon sauce   *1st Day Dinner*

1 tablespoon butter
1 tablespoon lemon juice
½ teaspoon dry mustard
½ teaspoon garlic powder
½ teaspoon marjoram
4 cups chopped, steamed broccoli florets

Melt butter and stir in lemon juice and seasonings. Stir well and pour over broccoli. *Serves 4.*

Roasted red peppers   *1st Day Dinner*

2 red peppers
2 cloves garlic, peeled and sliced
1–2 dashes olive oil
Salt and pepper to taste
Parsley sprigs

Preheat oven to 450 degrees. Roast peppers in oven, turning often. When skin covering pepper is black and puffy, remove from oven. Place in a double paper bag. Let cool for 2–3 minutes. Peel away burnt outer skin and remove seeds. The peppers will easily fall apart into bite-sized pieces; place these in bowl and toss with garlic and olive oil. Season with salt and pepper to taste. Garnish with parsley sprigs for a flavorful treat. *Serves 2.*

Fresh fruit shake   *2nd Day Breakfast*

1½ cups soy milk
1 ripe banana
½ cup frozen strawberries
Several ice cubes

Blend until mixture is thick and ice is crushed. *Serves 2.*

Raw vegetable salad with peanut sauce   *2nd Day Lunch*

½ medium-sized head romaine lettuce, chopped medium
   small
3–4 red radishes, sliced thin
2 scallions, chopped
1 tablespoon chopped black olives
Handful of fresh chopped parsley
2 tablespoons safflower oil
1 teaspoon salt
½ teaspoon oregano
½ teaspoon basil
Juice of 1½ lemons

Combine all ingredients and mix well. Top with Peanut
Sauce.

Peanut Sauce:

½ cup peanut butter
⅔ cup water
⅓ teaspoon salt

Combine ingredients and stir or blend until smooth, creamy
consistency is reached. *Serves 2–4.*

Guacamole spread   *2nd Day Lunch*

1 ripe avocado
1½ tablespoons lime juice
¼ cup minced onion
1 clove garlic, minced
¼ teaspoon cumin
1 small ripe tomato, finely chopped
1 tablespoon finely chopped green chili peppers
Dash of sea salt

Place meat of avocado in bowl. Mash lime juice into avocado
with fork. Stir in remaining ingredients. Chill guacamole and
serve at room temperature. *Serves 2.*

Broccoli-cashew tostada   *2nd Day Dinner*

3 corn or flour tostadas (large tortillas, available in the
    freezer section of food stores)
⅓ head broccoli, chopped and steamed
⅓ cup unsalted cashew pieces (may be roasted)
1 medium onion, minced and steamed
1 stalk celery, finely chopped
⅓ teaspoon chili powder
Handful of fresh coriander
½ teaspoon salt

Preheat oven to 325 degrees. Bake tostadas for 12 minutes,
turning once (6 minutes on each side). Meanwhile, combine
all other ingredients and mix well. Remove tostadas from
oven, spoon vegetable mixture on top and serve. *Serves 3.*

Sprouted-wheat and carrot bread   *3rd Day Breakfast*

1 cup wheat berries
¼ cup grated carrot

Soak wheat berries for 2 days, rinsing daily, until sprouts
barely pop through seed coats. Preheat oven to 200 degrees
(or lowest possible baking temperature). Combine sprouted
wheat berries with carrot; mix well. Spread mixture evenly
in 8 x 12-inch baking dish, and bake for 1½ to 2 hours. Enjoy
with your favorite nut butter! *Serves 6.*

Four-sprout salad   *3rd Day Lunch*

⅓ cup alfalfa sprouts
⅓ cup soy sprouts
⅓ cup mung bean sprouts
⅓ cup lentil sprouts
4–5 leaves romaine lettuce, chopped
1½ tablespoons sesame oil
1 tablespoon apple cider vinegar
1 tablespoon tamari (soy) sauce

Sprouting Instructions:
Wash 2 tablespoons each seeds or beans. Soak in wide-mouth jar as follows:

alfalfa	6 hours
lentil/mung bean	16 hours
soy	24 hours

Drain off water. Cover jar with cheesecloth and place in warm dark place. Rince twice a day and drain. After 3 days or when sprouts are approximately 1 inch long, they are ready to eat.

Combine sprouts and lettuce in large bowl. In separate bowl, combine oil, vinegar and tamari; mix well. Sprinkle dressing over salad; toss together. *Serves 2.*

Spicy onion-mushroom spread   *3rd Day Lunch*

2 tablespoons sesame or soy oil
1 large onion, finely chopped
1 cup grated carrots
1 cup chopped mushrooms
8 medium garlic cloves, finely chopped
8 ounces tofu
1 teaspoon rosemary
½ teaspoon thyme
2 tablespoons tahini (sesame butter)
2 tablespoons tamari (soy) sauce

Heat oil in wok or covered frying pan. Sauté onion until transparent. Sauté carrots until soft. Then sauté mushrooms and garlic until dark. Mash tofu and mix with other ingredients, stirring well. Add to wok and cook for another 10 minutes. Allow to cool, then blend in food processor or meat grinder. Refrigerate. Serve on celery stalks, crackers or whole-grain bread, or use as a dip for raw vegetables. *Serves 8.*

South American seviche — 3rd Day Dinner

3 fresh white-meat fish fillets
½ cup white wine
½ cup lemon juice
1½ Bermuda onions, thinly sliced
½ cup water
1 teaspoon salt
¼ cup apple cider vinegar
¼ teaspoon ground chili peppers or cayenne
Dash of pepper
3 tablespoons minced red bell pepper
3 tablespoons minced parsley
2 cooked sweet potatoes, sliced
Lettuce

Wash fish carefully and cut into thin strips. Place in bowl and add wine and lemon juice. Marinate at room temperature for 3 hours. Place onions in separate bowl. Add water and ½ teaspoon salt, and soak for 20 minutes. Pour off water and squeeze remaining moisture from onions. Rinse with fresh water and drain. Return onions to bowl and add vinegar. Soak for 1 hour, then drain. Add chili pepper, pepper, ½ teaspoon salt, bell pepper and parsley. Add fish. Mix together carefully and marinate in refrigerator 2 hours. Serve cold. Garnish with sliced sweet potato and lettuce leaves. (Also delicious served with salad of watercress, endive, cucumber and arugula.) *Serves 3.*

Wonderful Waldorf salad — 3rd Day Dinner

¼ pound apples
4 stalks celery, chopped
1 tablespoon lemon juice
Pinch of salt
2 tablespoons natural eggless mayonnaise
¼ cup chopped nuts
Pinch of pepper

Peel, core and dice apples. Mix with chopped celery, lemon juice and salt. Chill 1 hour. Stir in mayonnaise, chopped nuts and pepper. Serve on shredded lettuce. *Serves 3.*

Tropical fruit cup with creamy topping   *4th Day Breakfast*

1 kiwi, peeled and sliced
½ cup sliced mango
½ cup cubed fresh or canned unsweetened pineapple
½ sliced raw banana

Arrange fruit decoratively on dish. Pour on Creamy Topping.

Creamy Topping:

1 pear, peeled and diced
¼–½ cup water
½ cup cashews

Blend pear and ¼ cup water in blender. Slowly add cashews. Add more water if needed. Blend for several minutes until creamy in texture. *Serves 2.*

Avocado salad   *4th Day Lunch*

1 avocado, cubed
1 stalk celery, finely chopped
2 scallions, finely chopped
½ cup chopped lightly steamed broccoli
1 tablespoon soy oil
¼ teaspoon salt
Juice of ½ lemon
Small handful of watercress

Toss all ingredients except watercress in large bowl. Garnish with watercress. *Serves 2.*

Baked nut loaf   *4th Day Dinner*

½ cup cashews
½ cup sunflower seeds
½ cup blanched almonds
½ onion
⅔ cup cubed carrot
1 cup cubed zucchini
½ cup finely chopped celery
½ teaspoon basil
1 teaspoon tarragon
½ teaspoon powdered sage
2½ tablespoons arrowroot flour
⅔ teaspoon salt
2 tablespoons sesame oil

Soak cashews, sunflower seeds and almonds overnight in just enough water to cover. Preheat oven to 375 degrees. Steam onion, carrot and zucchini in stainless steel steamer basket until tender. Meanwhile, grind drained nuts in blender or food processor until mealy. Place in large bowl. Mince cooked onion in blender. Add all vegetables to nut mixture and grind to soft consistency. Add remaining ingredients and mix well. Spread evenly in greased 9 x 5-inch loaf or casserole pan, and bake for approximately 20 minutes. *Serves 4.*

**Colorful coleslaw with
vinegar-sesame dressing**   *4th Day Dinner*

⅛ head red cabbage, thinly sliced
⅛ head green cabbage, thinly sliced
½ teaspoon sea salt
¼ cup grated carrot
¼ cup diced celery
⅛ cup diced onion
Vinegar-Sesame Dressing*

Sprinkle cabbage with salt and let sit for 10–15 minutes. Squeeze the moisture from cabbage and rinse away remaining salt if desired. Combine cabbage, carrot, celery and onion in large bowl, and toss with Vinegar-Sesame Dressing.

Vinegar-Sesame Dressing:

1 tablespoon rice or cider vinegar
1 tablespoon light or dark sesame oil

Mix well. Use only enough dressing to moisten salad. *Serves 2.*

Mixed sprouts and tofu   4th Day Dinner

Sprouts: alfalfa, lentil, chickpea, mung bean
4 ounces tofu cake, cubed

Sprouting Instructions:
Wash 2 tablespoons each seeds or beans. Soak in wide-mouth jar as follows:

alfalfa	6 hours
lentil/mung bean	16 hours
chickpea	24 hours

Drain off water. Cover jar with cheesecloth and place in warm dark place. Rinse three times a day and drain. After 3 days or when sprouts are approximately 1 inch long, they are ready to eat.

Add tofu to mixed sprouts. Top with lemon juice and olive oil. *Serves 3.*

Tropical "smoothie"   4th Day Snack

½ papaya
½ banana
2 ounces pineapple chunks
1 cup crushed ice

Blend together in blender. *Serves 2.*

Salmon spinach salad   *5th Day Lunch*

4 ounces fresh salmon
Pinch of dill (optional)
2 cups spinach
1 small red onion
5–6 black olives
Juice of 1 orange
½ teaspoon honey
1 teaspoon tarragon
½ teaspoon sea salt
1 tablespoon olive oil
½ cup alfalfa sprouts

Poach salmon in small amount of water (barely enough to cover fish). Season water with dill and pinch of sea salt if desired. Chill. Wash spinach carefully and remove stems. Chop spinach, onion and olives. Break salmon into bite-sized pieces. Combine with other ingredients and mix well. *Serves 2–3.*

Light tabouli salad   *5th Day Dinner*

½ cup dry bulgur (cracked wheat)
1 cup hot water
1 medium onion, chopped, *or* ½ bunch scallions, chopped
⅓ cup chopped mint leaves
1 cup chopped parsley
½ cup chopped tomatoes
2 tablespoons soy or olive oil
Juice of 1 lemon
⅓–½ teaspoon salt

Soak bulgur in hot water until grains become fluffy; drain excess water. Add remaining ingredients and mix well. *Serves 3.*

Great gazpacho

¾ pound tomatoes
½ onion
½ cucumber
½ green pepper
1 cup water
1 cup tomato juice
1 tablespoon wine vinegar
½ tablespoon olive oil
Pinch of sea salt
Pinch of black pepper
2 cloves garlic, minced

Peel and chop tomatoes and onion. Peel, seed and chop cucumber. Seed and chop pepper. Puree *half* of the tomatoes, onion, cucumber and green pepper with water. Pour in large bowl; add tomato juice, vinegar, oil, salt, pepper and garlic. Refrigerate for 2 hours. Add remaining vegetables just before serving. *Serves 4.*

Tossed delight salad

¼ cup shredded romaine lettuce
¼ cup shredded red and green leaf lettuce
¼ cup shredded green cabbage
⅛ cup chopped onion
1 scallion, sliced
⅛ cup finely diced red pepper
1 teaspoon salt

Mix all ingredients. Place in salad press or in large bowl with a plate covering the salad and a weight on top of the plate. Let stand for about 2 hours. Drain excess liquid and rinse off excess salt. Season with chopped basil and parsley. Toss with a light dressing of cider vinegar and sesame oil. *Serves 2.*

Baba ghanoush *6th Day Lunch*

2 medium eggplants
¼ cup tahini (sesame butter)
¼ cup minced onion
¼ cup fresh lemon juice
1 clove garlic
¼ teaspoon cumin
1 tablespoon olive oil
1 tablespoon minced parsley
¼ teaspoon paprika

Broil eggplant at 375 degrees for 10 minutes. Turn over and pierce skin on top of eggplant with fork. Continue broiling another 10 minutes until skin on all sides is charred. Remove from broiler and let cool. Cut in half lengthwise and scoop pulp into bowl. Mash all ingredients into eggplant, cover and refrigerate. Serve on romaine leaves. *Serves 4.*

Cold pasta salad *6th Day Dinner*

8 ounces whole-wheat, corn or rice pasta
2 scallions, chopped
1 medium carrot, grated
1 small piece fresh ginger, finely minced
2 tablespoons dark sesame oil
1 tablespoon tamari (soy) sauce
2 tablespoons tahini (sesame butter)

Boil pasta as directed, drain and rinse with cold water in colander. Sprinkle in scallions and carrot. Add remaining ingredients and mix well. Serve with endive and escarole dressed with lemon and minced garlic. *Serves 4.*

Special herbed potato salad
6th Day Dinner

2 cups cold diced cooked potatoes
4 ounces tofu, diced
2 tablespoons parsley
Dash of pepper and salt
½ teaspoon dill
1 tablespoon chives, chopped
1 tablespoon apple cider vinegar

Mix ingredients well. Serve over lettuce. *Serves 6.*

Cold zucchini salad
7th Day Lunch

1 medium-sized zucchini, sliced into rounds
1 clove garlic, minced or sliced
Salt and pepper to taste
1 teaspoon olive oil
1 tomato, sliced into wedges
Fresh basil leaves, chopped, to taste
Fresh dill, chopped, to taste
Dash of tarragon vinegar (optional)

Sauté zucchini, garlic and a pinch of pepper in olive oil. After cooking 5 minutes, add tomato, basil and dill. Continue sautéing 5 minutes more. Use a dash of tarragon vinegar for added flavor. Chill. Serve with thin wheat or rye crackers. *Serves 3.*

Sesame bluefish stuffed tomatoes
7th Day Dinner

Sesame Bluefish:
6 ounces bluefish
1 tablespoon tamari (soy) sauce
1 tablespoon water
2 tablespoons sesame oil
1–2 ounces sesame seeds

Preheat oven to 425 degrees. Place fish in baking pan. Combine tamari with water, stir in oil and pour over fish. Turn fish in liquid to coat all sides; sprinkle with sesame seeds. Bake for 8–9 minutes or until tender.

4 large tomatoes
6 ounces Sesame Bluefish, mashed
2 scallions, chopped
1 green pepper, chopped
¼ teaspoon oregano
¼ teaspoon marjoram

Slice off tops of tomatoes and scoop out insides. Mix cooked bluefish with scallions, green pepper and seasonings. Carefully stuff into tomato skins. Serve on a bed of lettuce. *Serves 4.*

Vegetables marinade   *7th Day Dinner*

2 tablespoons honey
¼ cup apple cider vinegar
2 tablespoons peanut oil
¼ cup tahini (sesame butter)
½ teaspoon salt
¼ teaspoon dry mustard
¼ teaspoon dill weed
¼ teaspoon marjoram leaf
¼ teaspoon allspice
¼ cup cooked adzuki beans (small red beans available from
    health-food stores) or adzuki bean sprouts
½ cup finely chopped broccoli
½ cup sunflower seed sprouts
½ cup finely chopped cauliflower

Combine honey, vinegar, oil, tahini and seasonings. Mix well. Toss marinade onto vegetables, beans and sprouts. Cover and refrigerate overnight. *Serves 3.*

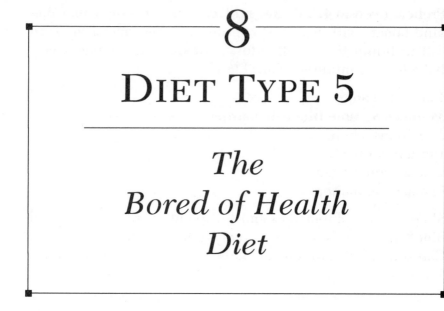

8

DIET TYPE 5

The Bored of Health Diet

A good friend of mine regards hamburgers as an American institution. Whenever I urge him to try an occasional soybean "burger" or maybe stir-fried vegetables with tofu, he looks at me with horror, as if I were suggesting something subversive. Though he wouldn't admit it, I think he'd feel positively unpatriotic or out of his element if he took to eating any "exotic" meal too often. Another friend can't seem to shake her habit of carting home a fast-food lunch or dinner whenever she's in a hurry (and that turns out to be almost every day!). After years spent coaxing and trying to change their eating habits, as well as those of many of my own dieting patients, I decided instead to design a healthful eating plan based on their idiosyncrasies and not-so-wholesome habits.

That's what led eventually to the Bored of Health Diet, or Type 5. It's aimed primarily at those who can't or don't want to rely on grain- or vegetable-based meals or who don't live in places where such foods are easily available. They have little time or interest when it comes to cooking or planning menus and prefer quick take-out shops or packaged super-market foods—in other words, standard American fare. Maybe they want to relax and indulge in the familiar "fun" foods they associate with childhood rather than be nutrition-conscious all the time. Or perhaps they don't mind counting calories and are frankly bored with health food.

Other people might adopt this diet more out of necessity than choice. They travel for their jobs so often that they're dependent on restaurant or roadside meals. The Bored of Health Diet can also serve as a strictly temporary strategy for the already conscientious eater. If you're at a holiday party or having dinner at an aunt's, for example, how can you enjoy your meal and maintain your diet, too?

The foods on this all-American menu are easy to find and prepare—no bean-soaking or pressure-cooking required!—and adapt readily to travel. This down-to-earth program also *desensationalizes* dieting, taking some of the fuss and atten-tion away from the whole process of slimming down.

On the downside, this kind of diet may sometimes leave you prey to undesirable ingredients. For example, a number of "lite" products that purport to be lower in calories are often not much better than the originals; they may still be unacceptably high in salt, hydrogenated fats and cholesterol, and low in fiber. Other low-calorie foods that are sweetened artificially may stimulate the appetite and trigger an insulin response that can leave you hungry soon after eating. Studies have suggested that part of the insulin mechanism may be cerebral, meaning that even a sweet-tasting chemical may have the same physiological effect as sugar.

Another drawback is that in its popular form, this way of eating does not give you maximum protection from certain major diseases. One of my patients recently reported that she had lost over 25 pounds and had "never felt better" on this kind of diet. Her daily menus relied heavily on Lean Cuisine dinners, canned soups, frozen vegetables and other packaged convenience foods (she was arthritic and had difficulty preparing more than simple meals). However, when I checked her, I found her tryglyceride levels alarmingly high. Because her father had had a major heart attack at fifty, I felt she would be at considerable risk unless I intervened. Her low-calorie meals had enabled her to drop all her unwanted weight. Why, then, did her blood profile tell a different story? She was on a Bored of Health type of diet all right, but her choices were hit-or-miss—too high in fat, too low in fiber, and the combination had sent her blood fat levels soaring. She needed the proper guidance on how to put her convenience meals together in a way that maximized not only weight loss, but also her personal health and longevity.

Drawing on the latest nutritional know-how, I have developed this Diet Type for both efficient weight loss and optimal health. Included are guidelines for strategic supermarket shopping and for eating slim and smart even if you're a fast-food junkie or are convinced that all products labeled "lite" are right for you. If you can't live without red meat, you'll learn how to build a safer and leaner menu plan around it.

As it stands, the typical American diet is still extravagant when it comes to sugar, fat, salt, cholesterol and other saboteurs of both slimness and health. If you're a diehard champion of the staples of American cuisine and refuse to give them up, the good news is that you don't necessarily have to. Using these items is largely a matter of degree, and fortunately a little of each can go a long way toward pleasing your palate without adding unwanted calories or endangering your health. With a few gradual, strategic substitutions, you can free yourself of your overdependence on the most tempting ingredients, and ultimately you'll find you "need" very modest amounts, if any, to appease your hunger and satisfy you.

You'll be surprised at how many recipes or restaurant meals can be modified with a bit of easy planing, without noticeably altering their texture or taste. Lower-calorie counterparts are readily available, some a lot better (and more delicious) than others. The simple secret is to choose discriminately.

SUPERMARKET SMARTS

Thanks to consumers' demands, "lite" versions of almost every conceivable food are now stocking supermarket shelves and freezers. The latest surveys show that over twice as many people now follow a low-sodium regimen as did just five years ago, and four times as many are trying to control their intake of saturated fat. Not long ago, the only diet-wise items were skim milk, yogurt and sugar-free soda. Now meats trimmed of over half their fat, described as "lean" or "ultra-trim," cheeses with reduced cholesterol or salt, syrups with less saturated fat and sugar, low-sodium breakfast cereals, white bread with added fiber and less fat, and even more wholesome potato chips have joined the still-growing ranks in the "lite" revolution. And this doesn't count the already ambitious range of nutritious yet slimming choices at the best health-food stores and greengrocers shops. More on these elsewhere, however; right now, we'll focus on the great American supermarket, where the overwhelming majority of those who are "bored of health" still shop.

While the abundance of "lite" foods makes it easier to lose weight and stay trim, be aware that this label does *not* automatically assure a nutritious meal. Since few uniform regulations currently exist, a product described as lite may be lighter than its original only in color or texture. Some manufacturers use the term when they have simply reduced the size of individual servings. What all this means is that choosing the right lite food is a matter of reading a label's fine print. Make sure the product has substantially less salt or fat or significantly fewer calories than the regular version. Also, be sure that in exchange for less fat or sugar, you're not getting undesirable extras like added salt or saccharin—a common practice to make up for missing flavor.

Some more pointers: While "low calorie" means that a food contains no more than 40 calories a serving, the term "reduced calorie" tells you nothing about how a product compares to the standard version. Since there is no minimum number of calories that must be eliminated, the product could still be fattening. Moreover, while it may not contain table sugar (sucrose), it could be high in other, equally caloric sweeteners, such as dextrose or maltose (corn and malt sugars). In fact, the suffix *-ose* is always a tip-off to added sugar.

Another ingredient to watch for is polyunsaturated fat, especially in the form of hydrogenated or partially hydrogenated vegetable oil. Everyone knows by now that saturated fats are a major villain, but few of us are aware that polyunsaturates pose a health risk, too. Recent studies have shown that a diet rich in these omnipresent oils promotes cancer growth in animals (see also page 37.) While they lower cholesterol, they may still directly harm the delicate arterial walls, promoting arteriosclerosis. Furthermore, when the polyunsaturates are hydrogenated to any extent, they form compounds that may actually increase the risk of degenera-

---

HYDROGENATED OILS: THE HIDDEN HAZARD

We all need a small amount of unsaturated vegetable oils in our diet, since these are the major components of our cell membranes, helping, among other things, to regulate their fluidity, permeability and resistance to toxins and infectious agents. Until about the 1940s, the unsaturated fats that came from our diets and formed our cell membranes were in their natural state, all liquids at room temperature. But today's widespread use of hydrogenation to make margarines, vegetable shortenings and countless other food products can subject these oils to high temperatures and pressures, slightly altering their chemical structure. Some studies have shown that this can impair the function of cell membranes and make them more permeable to cancer-causing compounds.

tive disease; the body also metabolizes them differently from other fats, and it's their long-term, little-known effects that many scientists fear. Many processed foods contain palm-kernel or coconut oil, which are fully as saturated as common lard derived from animal fat. The process of hydrogenation adds to their danger, turning them into synthetic compounds that have only recently entered the food chain.

How, then, should you react to products listing "partially hydrogenated vegetable oil" among their ingredients? According to the Center for Science in the Public Interest (CSPI), the answer is *warily:* "Hydrogenation may be thought of as a 'wild card' because it adds uncertainty to food labels. And the vague term 'partially' only adds to the confusion. These uncertainties are increased by 'and/or' labeling regulations which permit manufacturers to state that their products 'may' contain 'one or more of the following oils' . . ."

Bored of health types, both plain, no-nonsense eaters and rich-food-loving connoisseurs, generally prefer butter to margarine—and I have no argument with them. But my reasons have less to do with taste than with ingredients. It's better to have a quarter or half pat of butter on toast or a baked potato than to swallow two whole pats of a product that's loaded with potentially carcinogenic polyunsaturates, along with artificial coloring and flavoring. Margarine is a synthetic food, and people often wind up eating too much of it in the misguided belief that it's actively beneficial to health or can significantly lower cholesterol—both untrue! The same holds for polyunsaturated cooking and salad oils. Despite seductive TV ads that suggest these play a major role in curbing heart disease and high cholesterol, in fact it's the monounsaturated, extra-virgin olive oils that do far better in this category, *without* posing any cancer risk. For those who think olive oil is too strongly flavored, remember there are a number of different kinds to choose from, including Spanish, Italian and French varieties, along with new "lite" versions that may be easier on the palate. If you do prefer corn, safflower, cottonseed or soybean oil, try to find one that's "cold-pressed"—meaning that it has not been heated and chemically altered, as the latter process could make it more subject to rancidity, or spoilage. Spoiling can lead to the formation of "free radicals," harmful compounds that do damage to the body's cell membranes, making them more vulnerable to carcinogens.

A commonsense Bored of Health rule is to avoid all processed foods that are high in fat. Unfortunately, this strategy is often easier said than done. While the labels on mayon-

---

LABEL LOGIC

On a label, ingredients are listed in the order of their weight, from highest to lowest. If you're trying to limit salt, fat or sugar, for example, avoid products that list these among their first few ingredients.

Sugar added to food has many names:

> dextrose
> fructose
> glucose
> honey
> maltose
> molasses
> sucrose
> syrups

A food contains *sodium* if its ingredients include the words "soda," "salt" or "sodium."

For example:

> **INGREDIENTS**: Potatoes, vegetable oil, whey, *salt*, dried milk solids, sour cream, *onion salt*, *monosodium glutamate*, dried parsley, lactic acid, *sodium citrate*, artificial flavors.

Adapted from the U.S. Department of Agriculture.

naise, peanut butter and potato chips often state their saturated and polyunsaturated fat contents, few other products furnish this information. (Only slightly more than half of all labels list total fat content.) In some cases, you may be able to estimate how much fat a product contains by scanning the list of ingredients, reading the labels on comparable products, or writing to the manufacturer.

While I certainly prefer it to margarine, butter is a potent source of saturated fat and cholesterol, so portion size is crucial. Bored of Health menus will feature no more than about half a pat on foods. The same goes for mayonnaise, sour cream, cream sauces and the like: If you think of them as dollop-sized garnishes, you can indulge in them all and still stay within reasonable calorie limits.

Instead of sautéing foods in butter, try a nonstick pan, or use equal amounts of butter and olive oil to reduce fat content and add healthful monounsaturates.

When shopping for fresh or prepared meats, look for the "lean," "low-fat" or "ultra-trim" varieties. This means the fat, sodium, cholesterol and/or breading has been cut by at least one-quarter. Chicken and turkey, of course, are already trimmer than red meats, with less saturated and more monounsaturated fat; some chicken producers, such as Perdue and Holly Farms, are now coming out with leaner-than-ever birds.

SHAKING OUT THE SALT

If you are feasting mostly on canned, packaged and frozen foods, beware of the omnipresent sodium. Fortunately, an increasing number of low-sodium alternatives are now available, and the FDA has also established strict labeling standards. Look for the following labels:

- *sodium-free:* less than 5 milligrams a serving
- *very low sodium:* 35 milligrams or less

BE ALERT!

The new "lites" are neither a guarantee of healthful eating nor a license to overindulge. Choose such foods carefully (check all labels) and make sure you have sensible portions. Portion control is indispensable to the success of the Bored of Health Diet.

- ▪ *low sodium:* reduced by at least 75 percent from the original product.
- ▪ *no salt added:* none added during processing

While most nutrition authorities currently recommend that our *maximum* sodium intake be within the range of 1,100 to 3,000 milligrams a day, for patients with a tendency toward high blood pressure, it's better to keep this amount well under 1,000 milligrams a day.

LESS SALT, STRONGER BONES?

One little-known reason to cut down on salt: it may reduce your risk of osteoporosis. A recent Dutch study reported in *Nutrition Action,* the excellent newsletter published by the Center for Science in the Public Interest (CSPI) in Washington, D.C., found that doubling the sodium content of a diet from 3,000 to 6,000 milligrams a day causes us to lose (excrete) about 20 percent more calcium from our kidneys. Since we consume on the average about 4,000 to 6,000 milligrams a day, we are probably losing a good deal of this bone-building mineral in the process.

Note: Instant grain cereals, such as quick oats, instant corn grits and cream of wheat, contain a substantial amount of salt even though the grains themselves are sodium-free in their natural state. Apparently, it is added in the process of making them instant, or ready-to-serve. Solution? Just soak these cereals for a few minutes, pour out the water and then cook, and you'll eliminate much of the salt. (Alternative solution: buy regular unsalted rolled oats.)

FOOD UNDER WRAPS

Not counting milk and bakery products, more than half of all American food is processed, that is, canned, frozen or dehydrated.

The sterilizing heat that protects the contents of a can from spoilage also destroys nutrients, and foods with the lowest acid content fare the worst. For example, canned tomatoes, high in acid, lose only about a quarter of their vitamin C and none of their vitamin A, while green beans, lower in acid, lose 80 percent of their vitamin C and nearly a quarter of their vitamin A.

When shopping for canned goods, look for any leaks, a sign of spoilage. Also beware of dents in cans, since these weaken their seams, allowing bacteria to enter. Bloating and bulging are especially ominous. They are caused by germs left behind by improper sterilization that can give rise to botulism, a potentially fatal food poisoning. Always store cans, along with bottles and packaged dry mixes, in the coolest and driest possible place—not in the cabinet above the stove or beneath the sink, but in a location away from excess heat or moisture.

Interestingly, the size of a container can make a nutritional difference. Think about it: The larger it is, the longer it takes to heat during sterilization, which means more nutrients are lost in the process. A giant, restaurant-sized can of peas takes almost twice as long to heat through at the cannery as a standard 16-ounce can, and thus provides fewer nutrients in the bargain.

Frozen foods are a better bet. Just before vegetables are frozen, they are heated, or blanched for several minutes to curb bacterial growth that cannot be prevented by freezing

---

SUPERMARKET SAVVY

Leni Reed, a licensed dietitian in Dallas with a master's degree in public health information, created what she calls the "supermarket savvy" tour because she found many people were confused and misinformed about nutrition. Designed to show consumers how to reduce fat, cholesterol and sodium and add more fiber to their supermarket purchases, the tours are two-and-a-half-hour aisle-by-aisle guided walks through stores. For those who can't do it in person, a new videotape, "Supermarket Savvy Video Tour," is available by mail order.

Besides showing how to find maximum nutrition for the fewest calories, it contains practical consumer advice, answers to commonly asked nutrition questions and guidelines for heart patients, diabetics, overweight people and senior citizens. Highlights of both the live and taped tour include a comprehensive listing by brand name of nutritious canned, frozen, packaged, bottled and fresh foods; easy-to-prepare recipes for the chosen products; an herb and spice cooking chart; a list of recommended cookbooks and a roundup of diet-minded area restaurants.

For more information, contact:
Supermarket Savvy
P.O. Box 25M
Addison, Texas 75001- 0025

---

alone. But because the heat exposure is so brief, frozen foods retain far more nutrients. A survey of seven food items by the U.S. Department of Agriculture showed that frozen vegetables retained an average of 47 percent more thiamine, 18 percent more riboflavin and 25 percent more niacin and vitamin C than their canned counterparts. If frozen foods begin to thaw—and this can happen starting at about 25°F—they will lose both nutrients and flavor. Lower temperatures can extend their shelf life, of course.

In the store, reject frozen packages that seem limp or wet to the touch, a sure sign of defrosting. Likewise, one that is coated with snowy frost or ice has thawed and been refrozen at some point since it left the packaging plant. Such a food will definitely be short on taste, texture and nourishment, and may even harbor bacteria.

Don't keep foods more than a few weeks in the freezer of a one-door refrigerator, since temperatures there will rarely go below 10° or 15° F; by contrast, foods in the freezer section of a two-door refrigerator can keep well for several months. In a separate household freezer, where the ideal temperature of 0° F can be maintained, foods will keep well for up to twelve months.

THE FIVE BEST "LITE" FOODS

Recently, the Center for Science in the Public Interest in Washington, D.C., saluted five "lite" foods as "Most Valuable" for their substantially reduced fat, sodium, sugar or calorie contents.*

Kraft Light Mayonnaise: By adding more water to mayonnaise, Kraft has cut the fat content in half and reduced the calories from 100 to 45 per tablespoon.

Philadelphia Light Cream Cheese: By diluting the cream with low-fat cottage cheese and skim milk, Philadelphia re-

* Reprinted by permission of *HealthFacts*, November 1986, Center for Medical Consumers, 237 Thompson St., New York, NY 10012.

WHAT'S A CUT ABOVE?

How do America's familiar—and favorite—snack foods rate nutritionally? If you can't resist them, which ones are you better off eating? Here are the differences in quality among the junk foods in greatest demand:

Potato chips are composed of roughly 60 to 65 percent potato and 35 to 40 percent oil. The thicker the slice, the less oil is absorbed and the more potatolike the taste. Nutrients present, albeit in modest amounts, include protein, calcium, phosphorus, iron, potassium and niacin, and even smaller traces of vitamin A, thiamine and riboflavin.

Popcorn is about 10 percent protein and only 3 percent fat, and consists largely of starchy carbohydrate calories (a source of fiber) and water. When popped, however, its fat content climbs because the corn absorbs some of the oil used in the cooking process. But it's still a good snack choice for the weight-conscious, since a cup of it has only 40 to 65 calories. Homemade is best, because poor-quality oils are often used in supermarket varieties. And the new wave of home air poppers has made oil-free popcorn easily accessible to anyone with an electric outlet.

Pretzels, a longtime American staple, have some modest nutritional value when they are made with enriched wheat, rye and malted barley flours.

Pizza, especially with mushrooms, anchovies, peppers and similar garnishes, can also be a nutritious choice. The cheese (sometimes part-skim, low-moisture mozzarella) provides good-quality protein, and the overall nutrient content may be similar to that of many vegetables.

duced the fat and calories by about one quarter and slightly increased the calcium, protein and riboflavin.

Kikkoman Lite Soy Sauce: Kikkoman cut the sodium by almost 40 percent, while maintaining "perfectly good flavor." One tablespoon of Kikkoman's regular soy sauce contains about 960 milligrams of sodium, and the equivalent amount of Lite Soy Sauce has 599 milligrams.

Wish-Bone Lite Salad Dressing: Thanks to a reduced oil content, Wish-Bone's chunky blue cheese, creamy cucumber and French dressings are only 15 to 30 calories per tablespoon, as opposed to the usual 70 to 80 calories.

Mrs. Dash Crispy Coating Mix: An amount that can cover a quarter of a chicken or two large pork chops contains only 5 milligrams of sodium. Onions, herbs and spices are used in place of salt—a welcome departure from the usual potassium chloride substitute that many find unpleasantly bitter.

THE FAST-FOOD REVOLUTION

It's become a national tradition: Of the millions of Americans who eat out regularly, nearly a third of them choose "fast food." Happily, this is no longer just the familiar quarter-pounder, fries and shake. Salad bars, baked potatoes, low-fat milk and whole-grain muffins, along with such ethnic, more wholesome favorites as pizza, chili and tacos, are becoming standard fare, with more innovations on the way. So if you find such menus appealing, it's now easier than ever to fit them into a diet or healthful eating plan. But just like the supermarket shopper, you need to choose with care.

First, the good news: according to a report from Consumers Union, a typical meal—consisting of a Big Mac, Whopper or Burger Chef, french fries and a shake—provides close to one-third of the average daily nutritional needs and about 85 percent of a woman's recommended allowance for protein. It also contains at least one-quarter of the RDA for thiamine, riboflavin, vitamin B-12, niacin, phosphorus, zinc and calcium.

The biggest drawback with most fast food, however, is that it is extremely high in fat, sodium, sugar and synthetic and refined ingredients. The "typical meal" above also provides about half the daily calories needed by the average woman —which means it doesn't leave much room to splurge at other meals. Fast foods are also generally low in vitamin A and certain B vitamins, such as biotin, folic acid and pantothenic acid, as well as lacking in fiber. Of course, these deficiencies can be counterbalanced at other meals with grains, vegetables and fruits.

While chicken and fish are usually good low-fat alternatives to red meat, in fast-food eateries just the opposite is often true. These breaded, deep-fried items have a high percentage of calories from fats, sugars and carbohydrates. Probably fried at too-low temperatures, they absorb much of the fat they're cooked in and are more harmful to your arteries and waistline than even the thickest all-beef burger.

Fortunately, roast beef sandwiches, available at Roy Rogers, Arby's, Hardees and other outlets, are much leaner than either hamburgers or fried chicken and fish fillets. (Roy Rogers's version is the trimmest, with only about 2 percent fat, while Arby's and Hardees are 13 and 14 percent fat by weight, respectively.) An increasing number of roasted, baked and broiled entrees are showing up on menus, too. Long John Silver's Baked Fish and Arby's Roasted Chicken Breast were favorably "reviewed" in a newsletter published by the Center for Science in the Public Interest. Consider some contrasts: The baked fish has 151 calories, while its batter-fried counterpart has 370. It also contains the equivalent in fat of less than a half pat of butter (amounting to only 12 percent of total calories) and only 361 milligrams of sodium, compared to the six-pat quantity and 1,234 milligrams of sodium in the fried fish. At Long John Silver's, you can also order corn on the cob and mixed vegetables for an uncommonly nutritious "fast" meal. Arthur Treacher's broiled fish has only 245 calories, and the chowder, made with low-fat milk, averages about 110 calories a serving.

Arby's Roasted Chicken Breast contains 254 calories, with a fat content equivalent to that of two pats of butter; when fried, the same size breast nearly doubles in calories and quadruples in fat! Other foods that made the CSPI newsletter's "best" or "honorable mentions" list include the Shrimp Salad from Jack in the Box (*without* dressing), with only 115 calories and a quarter pat of butter's worth of fat. (Warning: the dressing has enough fat to equal five to eight pats of butter, depending on the flavor.) While Wendy's multigrain bun is a breakthrough of sorts, 83 percent of its flour is still unbleached white. (The rest is a mixture of wheat bran, oats, soy, barley, rye, corn, rice and wheat gluten.)

Some frankly fried items can be diet-worthy, too. Six made-from-whole-chicken pieces, or "Tenders," at Burger King add up to 204 calories, and a drumstick dinner at Roy Rogers totals 117. Both Burger King's and Popeye's chicken "pieces" are made from real chicken breasts instead of processed chicken, which includes fatty, ground-up skin.

The advent of the salad bar has definitely redeemed fast food's image. Broccoli, dark leafy greens, red and green peppers, bean and alfalfa sprouts, tomatoes, cucumbers, carrots, chickpeas and three-bean salads are now available at Wendy's, Burger King and Roy Rogers restaurants. Such nutritional newcomers will supply some of the missing vitamins A and C, folic acid and fiber. But even here, you need to choose with care. "Dress" them sparingly, if at all, and skip the pickled or mayonnaise-laden items such as pasta salads and coleslaws, as well as the ones tossed with bacon strips, croutons and American cheese. Another sign of progress is the reduced-calorie salad dressing at Wendy's, Arby's and Roy Rogers. Like those found in supermarkets, these lower calories and fat by roughly half. (Just two tablespoons of regular French, Italian or blue cheese topping on an average helping of lettuce, cucumbers, mushrooms, alfalfa sprouts, broccoli, carrots and cauliflower can often *triple* the calorie content—from 80 to 240.

Keep in mind that you have some control over sodium content. Take french fries, for example. Ten of these delectables coated with a shake or two of salt and a tablespoon of catsup totals 370 milligrams of sodium; minus the salt and catsup, however, they come to a mere 2 milligrams.

To save the most calories, stick to the plain basic burger, or the one with everything on it minus the catsup and mayonnaise. A child's or junior's size has about half the fat and calories of the regular kind.

Thanks to quick-service restaurants, breakfast is back in style. But the much-touted egg sandwiches (typically on biscuits, muffins or croissants), dripping with melted cheese or teamed with bacon, ham or sausage, are alarmingly high in fat. Instead, try plain scrambled eggs (150 to 180 calories). An omelet with onion, green peppers and mushrooms (Wendy's omelet #4) has only 210 calories. Add an English muffin, with 185 calories, and orange juice, with 75 to 80 calories, for a well-rounded morning meal. At McDonald's, hotcakes with syrup but minus the butter are a satisfying, low-fat 390 calories.

A much better choice than hash browns or home fries, the baked potato, now a staple at several fast-food chains, is low in sodium (the toppings add all the salt, fat, and cholesterol) and contains 1,360 milligrams of potassium, 60 percent of the U.S. RDA for vitamin C, 15 percent for iron, thiamine and niacin and 6 percent for riboflavin. (Eat the skin for extra fiber.)

What's ahead: McDonald's is said to be testing a "lite Mac," made with a leaner cut of meat, less sauce and two buns instead of the standard three; also on their drawing board is a grilled, skinless "chicken LT" sandwich.

Above all, dining at fast-food places can be fattening because the *faster* you eat, the more likely you are to *overeat*. Since it takes twenty minutes for the appetite control center in your brain to relay the message that your stomach is full, a five- or ten-minute meal can easily put you over your usual calorie limit. You may not feel you've had too much until it's too late. So follow the Roy Rogers slogan and "slow down" —it may save you a lot of pounds!

On the Bored of Health Diet program, you'll choose from the basic food groups—vegetables, fruits, protein, dairy, grains and fats—and a group of optional extras. The mainstays will be convenience and supermarket items, many reflecting the best of the "lite" and fast-food alternatives available now. Though portions are carefully controlled, your food list will also include some usually forbidden fare, such as peanut butter, ice cream and wine. Calorie levels are high enough to ensure adequate amounts of vitamins and minerals. Because proteins, fats and carbohydrates are in good proportion, you'll lose weight at a safe, slow, steady pace of one to two pounds a week.

CHANGE YOUR PORTIONS

If you are a steak-and-potatoes person, try being more generous with the potatoes and stingier with the steak. Consider that a potato supplies vitamin C, fiber, iron, zinc and potassium, among many other nutrients, and "costs" only about 110 calories. A six-ounce serving of steak contains iron and some B vitamins, but the price you pay in saturated-fat calories, cholesterol *and* dollars, too, is far steeper.

For your weight's and health's sake, three servings of red meat a day are excessive; aim for no more than two servings and occasionally try for just one. Also, rely as much as possible on chicken, turkey, seafood, pasta and rice dishes as alternatives.

SODIUM FACTS: ABOUT CONDIMENTS

Watch out for commercially prepared condiments, sauces and seasonings when preparing and serving foods for yourself and your family. Many, like those below, are high in sodium.

Onion salt	Soy sauce
Celery salt	Steak sauce
Garlic salt	Barbecue sauce
Seasoned salt	Catsup
Meat tenderizer	Mustard
Bouillon	Worcestershire sauce
Baking powder	Salad dressings
Baking soda	Pickles
Monosodium	Relish
glutamate (msg)	

A SHOPPING TIP

Many manufacturers are introducing foods with reduced sodium. Examples of types of foods that are now available in low-sodium form or with reduced or no added salt include the following:

Canned vegetables, vegetable juices, and
  sauces
Canned soups
Dried soup mixes, bouillon
Condiments
Snack foods (chips, nuts, pretzels)
Ready-to-eat cereals
Bread, bakery products
Butter, margarine
Cheeses

(Continued)

(Continued)

Tuna
Processed meats

THE SALT/SODIUM CONNECTION

The link between salt and sodium may be a little hard to understand at first. If you remember that 1 teaspoon of salt provides 2,000 milligrams of sodium, however, you can estimate the amount of sodium that you add to foods during cooking and preparation, or even at the table.

Salt/Sodium Conversions
¼ teaspoon salt = 500 mg sodium
½ teaspoon salt = 1,000 mg sodium
¾ teaspoon salt = 1,500 mg sodium
1 teaspoon salt = 2,000 mg sodium

SODIUM CONTENT OF YOUR FOOD

This table shows the sodium content of some types of foods. The ranges are rough guides; individual food items may be higher or lower in sodium.

Foods	*Approximate Sodium Content (in milligrams)*
Breads, Cereals and Grain Products	
Cooked cereal, pasta, rice (unsalted)	Less than 5 per ½ cup
Ready-to-eat cereal	100–360 per ounce
Bread, whole-grain or enriched	100–175 per slice
Biscuits and muffins	170–390 each

(Continued)

Foods	Approximate Sodium Content (in milligrams)
Vegetables	
Fresh or frozen vegetables (cooked without added salt)	Less than 70 per ½ cup
Vegetables, canned or frozen with sauce	140–460 per ½ cup
Fruit	
Fruits (fresh, frozen, or canned)	Less than 10 per ½ cup
Milk, Cheese and Yogurt	
Milk and yogurt	120–160 per cup
Buttermilk (salt added)	260 per cup
Natural cheeses	110–450 per 1½-ounce serving
Cottage cheese (regular and low-fat)	450 per ½ cup
Process cheese and cheese spreads	700–900 per 2-ounce serving
Meat, Poultry, and Fish	
Fresh meat, poultry, finfish	Less than 90 per 3-ounce serving
Cured ham, sausages, luncheon meats, frankfurters, canned meats	750–1,350 per 3-ounce serving
Fats and Dressings	
Oil	None
Vinegar	Less than 6 per tablespoon
Prepared salad dressings	80–250 per tablespoon

(Continued)

	(Continued)
Foods	*Approximate Sodium Content (in milligrams)*
Unsalted butter or margarine	1 per teaspoon
Salted butter or margarine	45 per teaspoon
Salt pork, cooked	360 per ounce

Condiments

Catsup, mustard, chili sauce, tartar sauce, steak sauce	125–275 per tablespoon
Soy sauce	1,000 per tablespoon
Salt	2,000 per teaspoon

Snack and Convenience Foods

Canned and dehydrated soups	630–1,300 per cup
Canned and frozen main dishes	800–1,400 per 8-ounce serving
Unsalted nuts and popcorn	Less than 5 per ounce
Salted nuts, potato chips, corn chips	150–300 per ounce

Some Major Points About the Table:
Unprocessed grains are naturally low in sodium. Ready-to-eat cereals vary widely in sodium content. Some have no salt added at all. Others are higher in sodium than most breads.

Fresh, frozen and canned fruits and fruit juices are low in sodium. Most canned vegetables, vegetable juices, and frozen vegetables with sauce are higher in sodium than fresh or frozen ones cooked without added salt.

(Continued)

(Continued)

A serving of milk or yogurt is lower in sodium than most natural cheeses, which vary widely in their sodium content. Process cheeses, cheese foods and cheese spreads contain more sodium than natural cheeses. Cottage cheese falls somewhere between natural and process cheeses.

Most fresh meats, poultry and fish are low in sodium. Canned poultry and fish are higher. Most cured and processed meats, such as hot dogs, sausage and luncheon meats, are even higher in sodium because it is used during processing to preserve them.

Most convenience foods are quite high in sodium. Frozen dinners and combination dishes, canned soups and dehydated mixes for soups, sauces and salad dressings contain a lot of sodium. Condiments such as soy sauce, catsup, mustard, tartar sauce, chili sauce and pickles and olives are also high in sodium.

Many low- or reduced-sodium foods are appearing on supermarket shelves as alternatives to those processed with salt and other sodium-containing ingredients. Check the label for the sodium content of these foods.

(Information provided by the U.S. Department of Agriculture)

SAMPLE MENUS

Beverages for all meals: herbal tea, black coffee or decaff, instant grain coffee (e.g., Caffix), skim milk, soy milk, seltzer, plain or sparkling mineral water, fresh vegetable juices or filtered tap water.

Dressings for salads: fresh lemon or any low-fat dressing; vinegar with 1 teapoon olive oil

Note: Use fresh fruit and vegetables as often as possible.

DAY 1:

Breakfast

1 slice Aunt Jemima Cinnamon French Toast with Poiret Apple and Pear Spread or Sorrell Ridge Conserves (fruit only)

Lunch

½ cup Light n' Lively Low-fat Cottage Cheese (1% Milkfat) on romaine lettuce

Sliced apples, grapes and pears

Dinner

1 serving Gorton's Light Recipe (260 calories) frozen fish

White Rose Frozen Peas

Bird's Eye Frozen Spinach

Snack

¾ cup plain Dannon Low-fat (1 percent) Yogurt with sliced fresh fruit

DAY 2:

Breakfast

1 soft-boiled egg

6 ounces Welch's Orchard juice

1 slice Pepperidge Farm Very Thin Multi-Grain Bread, toasted

Lunch

1 cup canned Barley and Mushoom Soup

Salad

1 slice Bran'nola High Fiber Dark Wheat Bread

Dinner

1 serving Benihana Chicken in Spicy Garlic Sauce

Green Giant String Beans

Salad

Snack

Chico San Rice Cake with 2 teaspoons Skippy Peanut Butter (creamy or chunky)

DAY 3:

Breakfast

⅓ cup H-O Cream Farina with ½ cooked apple, sliced
Skim milk

Lunch

1 slice Dorman's Light Natural Swiss Cheese on Ryeola Whole Grain Black Bread grilled with tomato, onion and cucumber slices and herbs

Dinner

1 Serving Uncle Ben's Country Inn Savory Brown Rice with Vegetables *or* Middle Eastern Lentil Pilaf Mix

Salad

⅔ cup fresh or frozen squash

Snack

Axelrod's Easy-Dieter Vanilla Low-fat Yogurt with 1 teaspoon each sliced almonds and raisins

DAY 4:

Breakfast

⅔ cup Nutri-Grain Corn cereal with ½ cup skim milk and 1 tablespoon Kretschmer Wheat Germ

Lunch

4 ounces Chicken of the Sea Dietetic Very Low Sodium Tuna on bed of greens

1 Sahara Mini Whole Wheat Pita

Dinner

½ cup pasta with marinara sauce

Salad

Frozen or fresh cooked carrots

Snack

4 Low Salt Wheat Thins *or*
2 Kavli Norwegian Crispbreads with Poiret Apple and Pear Spread

DAY 5:

Breakfast

⅔ cup Post Raisin Grape-Nuts with ½ cup skim milk and 1 tablespoon Kretschmer Wheat Germ

Lunch

1 serving Stouffer's Lean Cuisine Stuffed Cabbage

Fresh or frozen lima beans

Salad

Dinner

1 serving Weight Watchers Oven Fried Fish with Vegetable Medley

Salad

Snack

½ cup White Rose Frozen Whole Strawberries or Big Valley Frozen Freestone Peaches with ¾ cup Axelrod's Easy-Dieter Yogurt

DAY 6:

Breakfast

⅓ cup Wheatena with ½ cup skim milk

Sliced peach

Lunch

1 serving Stouffer's Lean Cuisine Tuna Lasagna with Spinach Noodles and Vegetables

Salad

Dinner

1 serving Stouffer's Lean Cuisine Breast of Chicken Marsala

Carrots

Peas

Snack

4 Low Salt Triscuit crackers with ½ ounce Dorman's Natural Low Moisture/Part Skim Mozzarella (1 slice)

DAY 7:

Breakfast

⅓ cup H-O Quick Oats

½ cup skim milk

Handful of raisins

Pinch of cinnamon

Lunch

1 serving Weight Watchers Chicken à la King

Salad

Fresh or frozen peas

Dinner

1 serving Stouffer's Lean Cuisine Oriental Beef with Vegetables and Rice

Salad

Snacks

1 cup Columbo or Weight Watchers nonfat vanilla
yogurt

2 Lorna Doone Cookies *or* 2 Sunshine Ginger Snaps

EATING-OUT SUGGESTIONS

AMERICAN:

Breakfast Choices:
Whole-grain toast
Poached or boiled egg
Oatmeal with skim milk
Shredded wheat or high-fiber cereal with skim milk
Fruit cup without syrup
½ cantaloupe or melon
Vegetarian omelet (vegetable, Spanish, onion, spinach or
    mushroom)
Grape-Nuts cereal with low-fat milk

Lunch Choices:
Salad with water-packed tuna or salmon
Soup and salad
Sandwich (white-meat turkey, tuna or chicken) on whole-
    wheat bread with lettuce and tomato
Salad-bar fixings
Plain baked potato and salad

Dinner Choices:
Turkey, chicken or fish with salad and vegetables
Baked potato (skip gravy, stuffing, sour cream)

Note: Fast foods are mostly fried. Stick with the salad bars
and use dressings sparingly.

CHINESE:

Request "light" dishes low in oil, cornstarch and sugar.
Avoid pork.
Vegetables with chicken and plain brown rice (instead of white or fried rice)
Bean curd with vegetables
Stir-fried vegetables
Moo Shu vegetables
Chicken in black bean sauce with vegetables

GREEK:

Greek salad with feta cheese
Moussaka

INDIAN:

Curried vegetables with rice and dahl
Chicken tandoori and vegetables
Flat breads
Basmati rice

ITALIAN:

Pasta primavera with salad
Skinless breast of chicken in wine sauce with salad
Broiled fish with pasta and salad
Escarole or broccoli in garlic sauce
Spaghetti with tomato sauce
Minestrone soup
Melon and prosciutto

JAPANESE:

Soba noodles with vegetables
Miso soup
Raw tuna sashimi
Nori rolls
Pickled radish

Sukiyaki
Udon noodles
Salmon or chicken teriyaki

MEXICAN:

Tostadas
Guacamole with tortillas
Corn tortillas with beans and vegetables
Spanish rice and beans
Chicken enchilada
Refried beans
Chili
Seviche

MIDDLE EASTERN:

Tabouli salad
Falafel
Hummus salad
Stuffed grape leaves
Couscous
Baba ghanoush (eggplant)

9

How to Stay Slim On Any Diet

No matter what their diet type, my overweight patients share the same goal: to lose pounds steadily and safely, with results that last a lifetime. Those who aren't burdened with extra weight are concerned primarily about eating for maximum health and energy and to protect themselves from illness.

No matter which category matches you best, if you're a serious dieter you may benefit from the strategies highlighted here. As you may recall from Chapter 2, fat cells, setpoints and slower-than-average metabolisms may pose a challenge, but it's still your eating behavior that counts above all, and you can definitely keep it under control!

The chapters on the Diet Types gave you all the basics, explaining how and why each one works, the ideas on which they're based, for whom they're most appropriate, their advantages and drawbacks and, of course, presenting the diets themselves—detailed eating plans with recipes and other guidelines you can implement right away. This chapter will tell you how to manage and stick with any of these diets and how to keep off the weight you lose. It will draw on the techniques and tips that I have tested and found successful in my practice and that my patients have shared with me. Take advantage of the collective wisdom!

It's well known that many people have trouble sustaining

TRUST YOURSELF

I have often noticed that dieters are not unlike the Victorians: virtuous and straitlaced to a fault, and very tough on themselves, yet also capable of rebelling in the most spectacular way. Rigid and rule-minded on the one hand, excessively indulgent on the other, they oscillate between two extremes and never learn to eat like ordinary people. By demanding more of themselves than is really necessary, they help pave the way for their own fall. (The tragic, pathological limits that dieters can reach are illustrated by anorexia and bulimia, two increasingly well-known eating disorders).

What makes dieters become fanatics? I think it's because they start out feeling so helpless and out of control. They believe they must resort to draconian measures to stay in line, or else they won't succeed. And by being so unreasonable, they virtually guarantee the failure they fear so much. In short, *they don't trust themselves.* If you can relax a bit and view yourself as a dependable, deserving person—someone who doesn't need constant surveillance—you are more likely to stay trim and healthy, and reasonably happy in the process.

Remember, self-trust is more important to weight loss than even the best-designed diet. In fact, don't bother starting a diet unless you have plenty of it!

weight loss for more than a few months. As one diet veteran has admitted, a feeling of panic overtakes her every time she loses a desired amount of weight and then tries to eat "like a normal person" again. "I guess I don't know how to relate to food the way naturally slim people do," she says. "Once I no longer have a diet 'safety net' to catch me, I fear losing control around certain foods and not knowing how much or how little I can have of something before it does me in." One of her obstacles is a lack of self-trust: She believes that without the discipline of a structured diet, she will soon resort to her former destructive habits. Another reason for her anxiety is that she has set unrealistic goals for herself and left little margin for human frailty. One slip does not mean she's unreliable or a weight-loss failure. If she learns not to expect perfect eating behavior she may not be so uneasy about managing meals on her own.

Also, contrary to what she might imagine, dieting and keeping off weight do not involve major sacrifices or radical lifestyle changes. And the differences between overweight and normal-weight people are not dramatic or irreconcilable. By comparing their habits and attitudes it's possible to identify the behaviors that lead to initial success with a diet and either reinforce or sabotage slimness. The following simple advice is based on such observations as well as the latest research in weight-loss science.

WHILE DIETING AND AFTER...

■ Set manageable, not overwhelming or perfectionist, goals. Aim to lose, say, five pounds in a month, not fifty within two months. You should also *expect* to have occasional setbacks or to be faced with temptations you can't resist. Knowing that you might fail every now and then can help keep you on course. You won't quit the moment you show you're less than perfect.

■ Some "self-talk" during weak moments often helps. Ask yourself what you want more: to eat fattening foods or to be slim and in great health, to look and feel terrific? And remember, the choice is not necessarily an either/ or, since you can and should give in to food urges sometimes. Eat part (no more than half) of the item(s), and discard the rest.

■ Keep track of what you eat. Do this whatever way is easiest for you, whether it's by keeping a list of what you eat and when, or by recording the information on tape. Many overweight people tend to eat unconsciously, automatically, and underestimate the amounts they actually consume. In fact, a surprising number of my patients who kept food diaries for a while admitted being surprised, even shocked, by how much and how often they ate. Only after you become fully conscious of your eating habits can you begin to modify them to your advantage.

■ Unlike thin people, the overweight too often eat *for reasons other than hunger*. Tension, anxiety, depression, habit, boredom and obsession with food are among the leading triggers. Eating can sedate you, shifting your focus away from overwhelming problems for a while. If you take the time to record what you eat, also note what you're feeling before, during and after the meal. If you can pinpoint when and why you eat for emotional satisfaction, you can start to work on replacing eating with some other mood-lifting or tension-relieving activity.

■ Just being conscious of your eating is effective. One nutrition clinic asked its patients to keep a food diary for a week. Two-thirds of them lost weight as a result of that activity alone—even though they had not been instructed to diet.

■ The best food diary would also note where and how you eat: Do you often stand in the kitchen, peering into an open refrigerator? Do you always taste food as you cook? Do you find yourself eating while you're lounging on the sofa, watching TV? This last activity heads the list of weight-loss saboteurs. Studies have shown that people who watch more than an average amount of television tend to be overweight. After all, it's strictly sedentary recreation, its food commercials are powerfully persuasive and it also lends itself to leisurely—and mindless—snacking. Whole boxes of cookies and other "munchies" have been known to disappear in front of that magic screen!

In fact, never eat while you are doing anything else, which includes listening to the stereo, working at your desk or talking on the phone, or you may very well overindulge. Set aside enough time for sit-down meals only. No one is too busy to eat this way; if you feel you are, you'd better reevaluate your priorities!

▪ Many people overeat primarily out of boredom: Seeing, smelling, preparing and tasting food are habit-forming diversions. While television can be a boredom reliever, it's unfortunately one that encourages eating. Choose an activity that can *substitute* for eating, that will keep both your mind and hands away from food. Have you ever heard the phrase, "I was so busy I forgot to eat"? I'm not referring to the kind of busyness that leads to *skipping* any of your three essential meals, especially breakfast (see below). This will only cause you to overeat later in the day, when calories are burned off more slowly, if at all. The body loses weight most efficiently when calories are distributed over the course of a day rather than consumed in just one or two meals.

I'm speaking about engaging yourself between meals in work (or play) that's so mentally absorbing you "forget" even to think about food until you're truly hungry. Or occupy yourself physically, with a brisk walk or run, an invigorating racquet sport or even some major chore around the house. (Anything physical will burn extra calories, too.) The fuller and more varied your calendar with activities that interest and challenge your mind and body, the less likely you are to be preoccupied with food. From your diary, you might be able to identify the moments you overdepend on food (if you follow any pattern at all) and schedule such all-out work or recreation for these vulnerable times.

WATCH OUT FOR FINGER FOODS!

One Saturday last summer, my wife and I were buying groceries in a suburban supermarket. We ran into a neighbor, who eyed our cart filled with fresh vegetables and fruits. Looking quizzically at the piled-high produce, she asked us where all our "finger foods" were. "What do you mean by finger foods?" my wife asked innocently, not having heard the term before. "You know," the neighbor responded, "the kind you eat with your fingers right out of the box while you're watching TV or lounging around with friends. I couldn't live without them!"

Sure enough, her cart was nearly overflowing with boxes of all sizes and shapes: crackers, pretzels, cookies, potato chips and every other wrapped-up, "handy" edible you could think of. In fact, I didn't see anything that wasn't in some type of plastic or cardboard container. Our neighbor also happens to be fat. Coincidence? You decide.

If you do most of your problem eating at home, keep your refrigerator and shelves stocked with foods that either don't tempt you to extremes or that can be overeaten without consequences. See the fail-safe snack list at the end of this chapter for ideas. You'll be surprised and delighted to find out how many foods fall into this "no consequence" category.

Perhaps you don't overeat at all—yet you're still overweight. You may have graduated from a few too many weight-reducing diets, each time losing all the pounds you wanted to, but ultimately gaining them back. After several such experiences you swear you can eat a carrot stick and still gain weight. You may be exaggerating only slightly. After all, with each successive diet, your clever body has learned to defend itself against the threat of lost pounds by slowing down the rate at which it burns calories. As you read in Chapter 2, we are still programmed to protect ourselves from famine even though such a response is no longer appropriate. So when we restrict our food intake, our body auto-

WHY DO YOU OVEREAT?

Studies have shown that many people eat primarily to fill their *mouths* rather than their stomachs. They view food as the perfect pacifier, especially when they're under stress, and the mere act of chewing brings emotional relief. Mealtime becomes a daily way of coping, and they eat compulsively, out of mindless habit rather than insatiable hunger. In the short run, very high-fiber, low-calorie snacks can be effective tricks on any diet, since these help satisfy oral urges. People can overeat crunchy crackers, unbuttered, airpopped popcorn and juice, unpeeled vegetables without gaining weight. Meanwhile, professional counseling or support groups can uncover the problems that underlie their compulsive behavior.

Some people become and stay overweight because they are sensation-seekers. Endowed with more-sensitive-than-usual taste buds, they require more flavor, intensity and variety from their meals. Their fixation on food is fueled by a constant quest for sensory satisfaction and their appetites are often strongly aroused by the thought or mere mention of food. How a meal looks, tastes and smells is all-important. Selecting foods for their colors, shapes, textures and aromas as well as nutritional value can give the palate all the attention it desires.

matically compensates for the shortage by holding on to its calories more tenaciously. Some people have better built-in "famine control" than others, which may explain why they appear to gain and maintain weight so effortlessly!

While the body definitely resists any change in the status quo, it need not have the last word. Your first step is to follow a diet that provides no *less* than 1,000 to 1,200 calories a day. Remember, the more you starve yourself, the more vigorously your body will fight back. Eat more like a normal-weight person and your system will respond accordingly. Avoid having more than 500 calories in one meal (women especially may have trouble metabolizing more than this at a given time).

The next step is to increase your activity level: Sustained, vigorous exercise, such as walking, jogging, cycling, swimming and rowing, accelerates the metabolism and keeps it high for several hours afterward. If you have been on the diet-go-round, your metabolic batteries are probably winding down and need recharging. Aerobic exercise not only quickens your calorie-burning pace, it also rejuvenates your heart and lungs, improves muscle tone and may even curb your appetite. It stimulates the production of hormones that raise the blood fat level and make you feel fuller, and promotes other hormonal and biochemical changes that favor the breakdown and release of fat cells. It lessens the amount of lean body mass lost during dieting, too.

Also, it releases endorphins, natural mood-restoring, pain-relieving chemicals. When these are circulating freely, you won't need to rely on food to feel "high." And you'll start feeling so good about your body, you won't want to feed it anything but the best possible fuel.

Even when you do everything right, expect to get stuck at a certain weight for a while; no one ever makes steady downward progress. To escape the familiar diet plateau, reduce calories—but don't go below the 1,000 minimum—and do more aerobic exercise. Also, drink water! Just as with calories, the body hoards fluid when it it not getting enough. So, while it sounds paradoxical, drinking plenty of water will

DIETING MAKES YOU FAT

Each time you lose and gain back weight, your body becomes a less efficient calorie-burning machine. You also lose lean body mass but gain back more fat. That means your body composition acually changes and you become flabbier with each successive diet!

discourage the bloating and puffiness that can show up as extra pounds on the scale. Having a glass of water before each meal will also help fill your stomach and quench your appetite.

Weigh yourself no more than once a week—and do so at the same time of day. Body weight fluctuates constantly and a daily obsession with numbers can prove discouraging. What's more, scale weight is often misleading. For example, lean muscle weighs more than fat. So even if you are losing flab and replacing it with firm, body-contouring tissue, you may not be able to see the results on the scale right away. There's usually a time lag between significant weight loss and its impact on the scale. Ironically, of course, this doesn't apply to the loss of water weight, which is the strictly temporary result of so many of today's quick-fix diets.

Complex carbohydrates and lean proteins are less likely to turn into fat than fat itself. Carbohydrates are more likely to be burned for energy; protein is more likely to be utilized as a structural material in the body. The calories from fat are the most easily and quickly stored. Fats also pack more calories per ounce. (For example, 4 ounces of canned tuna in water has 180 calories; 4 ounces of cream cheese totals 400. So if you must overindulge, you're better off having an extra helping of potatoes, pasta or fish than adding on a pat of butter.

New studies have found that fat may be overrated as a satiety factor. Experiments suggest that you're likely to eat again sooner after a high-fat meal than following one high in carbohydrates. One possible reason is that carbohydrates trigger an immediate rise in blood sugar, while fats are only slowly broken down into sugar, so there is no feedback system that would tell you when to stop eating.

For many people, counting calories is an abstract, tedious way of gauging how much to eat. It also reinforces the notion of "forbidden" and "allowed" foods—and the split can undermine your best efforts. The foods that are labeled off-limits may become irresistible and tempt you to overeat. Thus, instead of encouraging responsible, pleasurable eating, rigid meal plans may inspire frustration and loss of control. Measuring portions of food—or, better, learning to estimate them by eye—may be preferable. Some nutritionists even recommend counting bites. This way, you can eat almost anything; it's just the amounts you have to control.

Find out what a 3- to 4-ounce portion of your favorite entree looks like, or buy a small food scale. Indulge in any dessert you want, but just have three or four (slow) bites' worth. Learning to eat less of any food and/or to stop after several bites will help prevent you from feeling cheated (or tempted to cheat in turn). It will also encourage you to eat more like normal-weight people do: Experiments have shown that the overweight often don't know how to have "just a little" or when to stop eating, while their slimmer counterparts have built-in satisfaction signals that tell them when they've had enough. That's why the latter seem to be able to eat even the richest foods without putting on any weight.* Another difference is that overweight eaters typically *rush* through their meals. Since it takes twenty minutes for satiety signals to reach the brain, eating too quickly causes them to miss this natural cue and overindulge. Wolfing down meals also means eating to the point of stomach-stretching fullness rather than pleasure. By taking measured,

---

* The biochemical reason, related to insulin release, that some overweight people don't know when to stop eating is discussed in Chapter 2, page 32. Learning to eat small, frequent meals more slowly can help the insulin do its job better and stabilize both your energy and appetite.

well-paced bites, normal-weight people actually taste and savor their food more.

Some commonsense ways to slow down: Take small bites, sip water and/or put utensils down frequently throughout a meal; use small forks and spoons, or chopsticks; eat with friends or family, not alone; start off meals with soup. Try to identify the exact moment you feel satisfied. Pause for a few minutes after you're half finished; continue eating only if you're truly hungry.

When you eat is as important as how much. Ideally, breakfast should be your most substantial meal and dinner your lightest. Try not to eat at all after 8 or 9 P.M., when your metabolism is at an all-time low. In a study done at the University of Minnesota, people who were given a single 2,000-calorie meal in the morning lost weight; however, when they ate the same meal in the evening, they either gained weight or lost a good deal less. Your body is least likely to store fat calories when you're most active—during the day. To put it another way, when you wake up, you must start your body's calorie-burning furnace once again. Remember, its thermostat has been set on "low" for six to eight hours during your inactive, foodless sleep. That's why breakfast is important. If you skip it, your metabolism will not have been properly fueled, which means you are more likely to store some of the next two meals as fat.

DRINK UP!

Paradoxical, but true: the more water you drink, the less fluid your body will retain. Water weight can make a difference of up to five pounds on the scale. Filtered tap water, seltzer and bottled spring water are best. Club and diet sodas are unacceptably high in sodium.

By passing up meals, you might think you're saving on calories, but instead you're making yourself too hungry— which could put you out of control the next time you see food. Also, when you eat irregularly or wait too long between meals, your body may start conserving calories as if it were defending itself against possible deficit, so you'll find it easier to gain weight. Moreover, your blood sugar may drop too low if you space meals too far apart. This could tempt you to reach for a sugary snack, which will only send your blood sugar plummeting further. Not surprisingly, skipping the morning meal has the heaviest consequences. Research has repeatedly shown that people who forgo breakfast put on pounds more readily than those who eat three square meals a day or several smaller ones with well-timed snacks.

Because eating itself can temporarily raise the body's metabolic rate (it generates heat), having at least three meals a day means that calories are more likely to be burned than stored. If you're on a 1,000–1,200 calories-a-day diet, try eating no more than a third of your calories at dinner.

REMINDER

Eating large amounts of food at one meal may send hormonal signals to your fat cells that cause them to multiply faster. This creates more storage room for any fat you eat and could make it harder for you to lose weight.

Of course, sticking to scheduled meals does not mean eating out of habit rather than hunger. For example, if you have a bigger-than-usual lunch, don't sit down to your regular-sized dinner; adjust your portions according to what you really want or need at the time. In other words, eat in response to internal cues—how hungry you are—not external ones, such as the time of day, family or social pressures or even the sight of other people eating. The overweight are typically more influenced by such outside stimuli than are their thinner counterparts.

If you are overpowered by the sight and smell of food and eat even when you aren't hungry, your best bet is simple avoidance. For example, take a detour so you won't pass the bakery or pizza shop on your way home.

IT'S THE LITTLE THINGS THAT COUNT

Overweight often accumulates slowly, insidiously, the result of small habits that add up over time. But you can reverse the process with subtle, easy changes. If you prefer, *start with one diet goal at a time.* For example, first cut down on fat, the most concentrated source of calories: Have plain, low-fat yogurt laced with herbs and spices on a baked potato instead of sour cream or butter; add lemon or tomato juice, wine vinegar and fresh herbs to salads instead of oily, creamy dressing, bacon bits, croutons or cheese; instead of mayonnaise, try soft tofu blended with garlic, lemon juice and a dash of extra-virgin olive oil. Next, focus on sugar: Stop adding it to cereals and coffee; have pureed fresh fruit instead of jam on toast at breakfast (freeze it for a predinner sherbet), a baked apple instead of apple pie for dessert; watch for hidden sugars in canned and other processed foods; try cinnamon as a sugar substitute.

Bake, slow-roast, steam and stir-fry foods instead of frying them (anything breaded and fried doubles in caloric value); use less butter and oil when sautéing and add more wine, herbs and defatted chicken broth; eat more fish and less meat. Serve meals to your family *restaurant style:* on individual plates rather than open platters that encourage second and third helpings; let someone else clean up afterwards, too. Always shop with a list, without too much cash and on a full stomach. Add a brisk morning or lunchtime walk to your daily routine. And be prepared: Plan scheduled meals as well as what to eat should hunger overtake you unexpectedly.

Sometimes, one simple change in your eating habits can make a surprising difference. A patient told me that he lost a few inches of fat around his middle in just three weeks by giving up his nightly ritual of eating a slice of pizza before going to bed. I have found this weight-loss strategy especially effective for those who are moderately overweight. Most likely, it is one unwise practice, such as late-night snacking on a fattening food, that made them overweight to begin with!

While it entails no major sacrifice or change in lifestyle, each new "small" good habit can contribute to your success in a very big way.

EATING ON THE RUN

It's no secret that vacations and business travel often spell disaster for waistlines and sensible eating habits. Whether you're bent on idle pleasures or making deals at a breakneck pace, you're likely to overindulge. In fact, a recent study suggests that meals away from home can pose a considerable health hazard. According to Norge Jerome, a nutritionist at the University of Kansas Medical School, frequent fliers take in an alarming proportion of their daily calories from fat, and considerably less from carbohydrates and protein.

Travelers are typically treated to more than their fair share of calories because many restaurants rely heavily on sugars, oils and greases as cut-rate means of enhancing flavor. But Jerome's study indicates that unwise choices also make the difference. For example, she has found that when eating out, men often order oversized steaks (up to 16-ounce portions) with plenty of gravy or catsup and a baked potato topped with sour cream; their desserts are the standard cheesecake or apple pie à la mode. While women tend to eat more seafood and salad, the first is often fried and the second may come loaded with dressing and such high-calorie extras as bacon bits and cheese.

Despite all these temptations, you *can* choose more discriminately. The answer is to plan your meals ahead of time, the same way you would a sight-seeing itinerary or business agenda. Sybil Ferguson, founder and director of the famous Diet Center franchise, which has had consistently impressive results for people trying to maintain their weight loss, offers some excellent advice to those like herself who are constantly on the road and must make do with restaurant menus.

What are your best morning choices? For a wholesome balance of fiber, complex carbohydrates and low-fat protein, ask for fresh fruit (it's better than juice because it's digested more slowly), a serving of whole-grain bread or cereal such as oatmeal or cream of wheat, a cup of plain yogurt or skim milk, one poached or hard-boiled egg and black or brewed decaffeinated coffee without sugar. And avoid the ubiquitous "continental breakfast" with its white rolls, croissants and butter. These refined carbohydrates, sugars and fats are high in calories without much redeeming nutritional value, and provide only a short-lived surge of energy.

For lunch, start with a glass of bottled mineral water and a salad with plenty of greens and raw vegetables (eaten as slowly as possible) so you'll be reasonably full before you begin the main course. Ask for dressing on the side and use no more than a teaspoon or two. This "token" of flavor will keep you from feeling deprived, without adding any significant fat. Or better still, ask only for vinegar or fresh slices of lemon to squeeze on top.

At lunch or dinner, scan the menu for fresh fish or seafood that's broiled, baked, steamed or in a salad with lemon and dill; poultry (remove most of the skin before eating) or a roasted, grilled or stewed lean meat like veal, rabbit or lamb. If you're vegetarian, good protein-rich substitutes include beans and grains such as rice, millet, couscous, polenta and bulgur. A baked potato is fine, but top it with just a teaspoon of sour cream and half a pat of butter, or ask for herbs and plain yogurt if they're available. If you order pasta, avoid sauces made with cream or butter; generally, pasta primavera or with seafood is best.

Changing your usual mealtime behavior can also help keep your weight under control. For example, be more assertive with your friends or colleagues—talk them into trying the nearest seafood restaurant instead of going to the popular steak house—and learn to speak up to your waiter, as well. This means asking that your omelet be prepared in a nonstick pan without butter or milk, that your rainbow trout be broiled with herbs and lemon only. Another behavioral trick is to look over menus quickly; the less closely you study them, the less tempting their contents may appear. And when in a group, try to order *first* so you won't be swayed by others' choices. Also, talk to your companions during meals. Doing more socializing than eating will help take the spotlight off food.

Don't overlook your flight as a possible source of surplus calories. You might wish to ask for the low-calorie, fresh fruit or seafood menu when making your airline reservations. Most carriers need at least twenty-four hours' notice to honor special requests.

Whether you're on holiday or on a business junket, make a commitment to being active once you land—it's indispensable to staying trim. Rushing from one point of interest or conference to the next shouldn't count as part of your daily exercise; in fact, it can generate tension, which makes you more susceptible to heavy, off-hours snacking. Instead, schedule in some invigorating, aerobic, stress-releasing activity—spend about thirty minutes at least three times a week on it. Pack a jump rope (just five minutes of jumping is equivalent to one mile of jogging), use the hotel pool or spa (get on the stationary bicycle or the indoor track), run along the beach or walk briskly through town.

Enlist the support of at least one friend or family member with whom you can talk when you're feeling discouraged or on the verge of "blowing" your diet. Remember, you're set-

AS FOR ALCOHOL . . .

Think of it as liquid sugar and drink it sparingly, if you must. The driest wines and champagnes and all distilled spirits are the least fattening; sweet liqueurs, cordials and cocktail mixes are the most. For cocktail snacks, choose raw vegetables with just enough dip for flavor instead of the hot hors d'oeuvres; typically high in fat and salt, the latter are insidious because they're nibbled so casually, even absentmindedly, between drinks and conversation. If you insist on alcohol, try white wine spritzers or coolers with plenty of ice, and sip slowly. Nonalcoholic alternatives include seltzer, spiced tomato juice or sugar-free tonic water with a dash of lemon, as well as the new nonalcoholic beers.

ting a *lifelong* goal. Don't panic after an episode of overeating. In fact, binges often result from the frustration of failing to meet some unreasonable goal.

Weight-loss groups can also see you through weak moments or encourage your efforts. Many of them prescribe no set diet, but rather offer reinforcement and behavioral strategies that can prove useful with any eating plan.

Be doubly motivated: Keep slim for your health's sake, not just your appearance. Slimmer people do live longer and have lower blood pressure, cholesterol levels and cancer rates, as well as fewer heart attacks.

You can control what you eat, instead of letting it control you. Whenever you're offered (or see) something fattening, tell others or yourself, "I don't want that," rather than "I can't have that." This assertion builds confidence and helps you feel in charge of the situation, not deprived by it.

Positive reinforcement helps, too. Reward yourself with

some nonedible treat every time you forgo a fattening food, give up a longtime junk-food habit, lower your blood pressure or cholesterol through sensible eating or show any other signs of nutrition progress.

If you're cost-conscious, add up the price of the extra food you buy regularly, such as snacks, ice cream, etc. Determine how much money you'll be saving every week or month by crossing them off your list—what an incentive!

Visualization is an excellent motivator. Imagine yourself leaner, more active and energetic, eating satisfying, healthy foods. Keep in sight photos of a younger you or someone else who's slimmer and fitter than you are now, and aim to match that image.

Don't hide your fat under loose-fitting clothes; wearing snugger outfits will keep your excess weight visible, undeniable, until you can do something about it.

Visualize, even fantasize, about what you *can* eat freely and indulge all you want if you feel the urge.

Get a medical checkup to rule out any conditions—diabetes, heart disease or high blood pressure, for example—that might call for special care while dieting. Also, let your doctor know if you are taking steroids, thyroid pills or other medications that might affect the rate at which you lose weight and release excess fluid.

If your compulsive eating behavior is too persistent and deep-rooted to confront on your own, seek professional help. You can get a referral from a family physician, overeaters' support group or hospital.

HAPPY ENDINGS

Lasting weight loss and optimal health are achievable goals. Not long ago, after I called for my next patient, an attractive, slender young woman poked her head through my office door. Rechecking my schedule, I began to explain to this "first visit" that by some mixup she had slipped ahead of a long-time patient; then I quickly did a double-take.

"Cheryl!" I blurted out, "It's you!"

Before me stood Cheryl, who, at 135 pounds, was 80 pounds thinner than the unhealthy 215 pounds she was enveloped in when she first entered that door eighteen months ago. I recalled how she had complained of feeling miserable and knowing only failure when it came to losing weight. She had tried "too many diets to count" and could never manage to keep her weight off long enough to make a difference in her life.

I had followed Cheryl's progress closely for the first few months of her diet-type program, coaching and cajoling her, wondering if she would make it. There were heartbreaking setbacks at first, like when Cheryl came in with an incapacitating foot infection a week or two into the rigorous new aerobic exercise regimen I had assigned her.

"What happened?" I asked.

"Ever hear of shooting yourself in the foot?" Cheryl replied. "I 'accidentally' dropped a knife on my foot the other day—got so puffed up I can barely walk on it!"

After a few midcourse corrections, though, Cheryl's healthy weight loss campaign got underway in earnest and she became a less frequent visitor to my office. So much so that on the date of our reunion I checked to see when she had last come in—and it was a one-year anniversary! Knowing full well the impact her spectacular weight loss would have on me, Cheryl connived a bit and had her "before" and "after" photographs neatly juxtaposed in the chart which she now handed me: one picture was of a rotund, baggily costumed woman laughing self-consciously, the other a professional studio portrait of a confident, shapely, lean individual.

What had brought about the change? She had given up the futile and short-sighted idea of dieting, as I had suggested, and had found a way of eating and living that fit best with her tastes in food, her habits and lifestyle, her body's needs. Taking the pressure off herself, she stopped being obsessed with having to lose a given amount of weight in a week's or month's time, and took the long view instead. As she put it, "I started thinking about eating for my health's sake first, increasing my energy, being more active, trying to feel better and protect myself from illness—and weight loss just followed naturally from that." Most important, she emphasized, "I eat moderate portions of the right foods—and never find myself in a state of deprivation which would lead me to binge."

Once she had identified her diet type, found the right nutritional match and made a commitment to feeling good and staying healthy, the rest was remarkably easy. Happily, her experience is no exception. Following her example and finding your most compatible eating plan will ensure the same results for you.

APPENDIX

A POTPOURRI OF SLIMMING SNACKS

Recipes are provided for all dishes marked with an asterisk (*). To find them, consult the Index at the back of this book.

- Any fresh, whole fruit (a good mix with ½ cup plain low-fat yogurt or 1 ounce goat cheese)
- ½ cup fresh blueberries, strawberries, raspberries, grapes or cubed cantaloupe; 1 cup fresh cherries; ¼ cup pineapple chunks, fresh apricots or banana slices; 1 medium apple, pear, nectarine, plum, orange or grapefruit.
- Any fresh vegetable or leafy green/raw vegetable salad with Special Dressing*
- Light Tabouli Salad* ¼ cup
- Four-Sprout Salad* ½ cup
- Tuna Fish or Chicken Salad* ¼ cup, on Scandinavian flatbread
- Unsalted whole-grain crackers, soda crackers, pretzels or matzo with ¼ cup low-fat cottage cheese
- 1 slice corn, pita, sourdough, rye, whole wheat or pumpernickel bread or ½ bagel or 2 unsalted rice cakes with 1 tablespoon apple butter or fresh fruit spread
- 1 medium baked potato with fresh herb and yogurt topping
- 1 cup onion soup (no cheese)
- 1 cup vegetable bouillon
- 1 hard-boiled egg with paprika (try eating just the white)
- 1 cup air-popped, unbuttered popcorn with 1 teaspoon herb-seasoned olive oil
- 1 Oat Bran Muffin*
- 1 ounce (¼ cup) pumpkin, squash or sunflower seeds

- 7 medium fresh shrimp, raw oysters or cherrystone clams with lemon and fresh dill dressing
- 1 thin slice of turkey or cheese wrapped around your favorite raw vegetable
- ½ cup kefir
- 1 ounce goat cheese with rice or rye cracker
- ½ cup low- or nonfat yogurt with fresh fruit
- Frozen banana
- ½ cup or small jar chilled baby food dessert (low in sodium and sugar)
- ½ cup fresh applesauce
- See snacks for all five Diet Types

BEVERAGES:

- 1 cup herbal tea with lemon and a dash of honey
- 1 cup seltzer with fresh fruit juice
- Tropical Smoothie*
- ½ cup apple cider
- 1 cup skim milk
- 1 cup skim-milk Droste's hot cocoa
- 1 cup skim buttermilk
- 1 cup Fruit Shake*
- 1 cup High-Protein Shake*
- 1 cup vegetable juice
- 1 cup Green Water*

FAT AND CHOLESTEROL CONTENT OF COMMON FOODS

DAIRY PRODUCTS

	Total Fat (grams)	Saturated Fat (grams)	Cholesterol (milligrams)
Milk, Yogurt and Cheese:			
Milk, whole, 1 cup	8.1	5.1	33
Milk, 2 percent fat, with nonfat milk solids, 1 cup	4.7	2.9	18
Milk, 1 percent fat, with nonfat milk solids, 1 cup	2.4	1.5	10
Skim milk with nonfat milk solids, 1 cup	.6	.4	5
Yogurt, plain, low-fat, 8-oz. carton	3.5	2.3	14
Yogurt, fruit-flavored, low-fat, 8-oz. carton	2.4	1.6	10
Cottage cheese, creamed, ½ cup	5.2	3.3	17
Cottage cheese, 1 percent fat, ½ cup	1.1	.7	5
Cottage cheese, dry, ½ cup	.3	.2	5
Natural Cheddar cheese, 1 oz.	9.4	6.0	30
Mozarella cheese, part skim milk, 1 oz.	4.5	2.9	16
Pasteurized process low-fat cheese product, 1 oz.	3.0	2.0	5
Pasteurized process filled cheese food (low cholesterol)	6.5	.8	1
DESSERTS			
Vanilla ice cream, ½ cup	7.2	4.4	30
Vanilla ice milk	2.8	1.8	9
Frozen yogurt, ½ cup	1.5	1.0	6
Orange sherbert, ½ cup	1.9	1.2	7

MEAT AND POULTRY *(The trimmable fat contributes much of the total fat and saturated fat to meat.)*	Total Fat (grams)	Saturated Fat (grams)	Polyun-saturated Fat (grams)	Choles-terol (milli-grams)
Beef rib roast, choice grade, roasted, 2 oz.				
Lean and fat	22.5	10.8	0.4	54
Lean only	7.6	3.7	.2	52
Beef rump, choice grade roasted, 2 oz.				
Lean and fat	15.6	7.5	.3	54
Lean only	5.3	2.5	.1	52
Beef rump, Good grade, roasted, 2 oz.				
Lean and fat	13.3	6.4	.3	54
Lean only	4.0	1.9	.1	52
Ground beef patty, cooked, 2 oz.				
Regular	11.5	5.5	.2	53
Lean	6.4	3.1	.1	53
Extra-Lean	3.5	1.7	.1	52
Pork loin, lean, roasted, 2 oz.				
Lean and fat	16.2	5.8	1.5	50
Lean only	8.0	2.9	.7	50
Liver, beef, cooked with fat added, 2 oz.	6.0	1.7	.6	248
Liver, chicken, simmered, 2 oz.	2.5	.6	0	423
Chicken, roasted, 2 oz.				
Light meat with skin	6.2	1.7	1.3	58
Light meat without skin	2.6	.7	.6	48
Dark meat with skin	9.0	2.5	2.0	52
Dark meat without skin	5.6	1.5	1.3	53
Turkey, roasted, without skin, 2 oz.				
Light meat	1.8	.6	.5	39
Dark meat	4.1	1.4	1.2	48

FISH, BEANS, AND EGGS	Total Fat (grams)	Saturated Fat (grams)	Polyun- saturated Fat (grams)	Choles- terol (milli- grams)
Halibut fillets, broiled, 2 oz.	.8	.1	.3	35
Cod fillets, broiled, 2 oz.	.5	.1	.2	35
Tuna, canned, oil pack, drained, 2 oz.	4.6	1.2	1.0	37
Shrimp, steamed, shelled, 2 oz.	.9	.1	.4	117
Crab, cooked meat, 2 oz.	.9	.1	.3	57
Oysters, shucked, cooked, 2 oz.	1.5	.4	.4	36
Great northern or navy beans, cooked, ½ cup	.5	.1	.3	0
Canned beans with pork, ½ cup	.6	.1	.3	0
Canned pork and beans in tomato sauce, ½ cup	3.3	1.2	.3	5
Egg, large, 1				
Whole	5.6	1.7	.7	274
Yolk	5.6	1.7	.7	274
White	Trace	0	0	0

FATS AND OILS (Amounts given are for one tablespoon.)	Total Fat (grams)	Saturated Fat (grams)	Polyun- saturated Fat (grams)	Choles- terol (milli- grams)
Animal Fats:				
Beef fat	12.8	6.4	0.5	14
Chicken fat	12.8	3.8	2.7	14
Lard	12.8	5.0	1.4	12
Butter	11.5	7.2	.4	31
Vegetable Oils:				
Corn	13.6	1.7	8.0	0
Cottonseed	13.6	3.5	7.1	0

FATS AND OILS (Amounts given are for one tablespoon.)	Total Fat (grams)	Saturated Fat (grams)	Polyun- saturated Fat (grams)	Choles- terol (milli- grams)
Peanut	13.5	2.3	4.3	0
Safflower	13.6	1.2	10.1	0
Soybean	13.6	2.0	7.9	0
Mixed (mostly soybean and some cottonseed	13.6	2.4	7.9	0
Sunflower	13.6	2.4	6.5	0
Olive	13.5	1.8	1.1	0
Coconut	13.6	11.8	.2	0
Palm	13.6	6.7	1.3	0
Margarine:				
Hard (stick)	11.4	2.1	3.6	0
Soft (tub)	11.4	1.8	4.8	0
Vegetable shortening, hydrogenated	12.8	3.9	1.8	0
Salad Dressings:				
Mayonnaise	11.0	1.6	5.7	8
Mayonnaise-type	4.9	.7	2.6	4
Italian	7.1	1.0	4.1	0
Blue cheese	8.0	1.5	3.4	3
French	6.4	1.5	3.4	0
Thousand Island	5.6	.9	3.1	4

SNACKS	Total Fat (grams)	Saturated Fat (grams)	Choles- terol (milli- grams)	Sodium (milli- grams)
Cracker- and Chip-Types:				
Potato chips, 10	8.0	2.0	0	200
French fries, salted, 10 long strips	10.3	2.6	0	189
Corn chips, ½ cup	6.1	1.3	0	188

SNACKS	Total Fat (grams)	Saturated Fat (grams)	Choles-terol (milli-grams)	Sodium (milli-grams)
Popcorn, plain, 1 cup	.3	Trace	0	1
Popcorn, salted and buttered, 1 cup	2.0	.9	4	175
Butter crackers, 4	2.3	.8	0	142
Saltine crackers, 4	1.4	.3	0	140
Whole-wheat crackers, 4	2.2	.5	0	120
Pretzels, salted, 10 thin sticks	.1	Trace	0	51
Nuts and Seeds:				
Peanuts, roasted, salted, ¼ cup	17.9	3.9	0	200
Peanuts, dry-roasted, salted, ¼ cup	17.6	3.1	0	200
Peanut butter, 2 tablespoons	15.3	2.8	0	162
Sunflower seeds, roasted, salted, ¼ cup	16.8	3.2	0	196
Dessert-Type:				
Chocolate chip cookies, 2	4.4	1.3	8	69
Frosted brownie, 1	6.6	2.2	12	69
Gingersnaps, 2	1.2	.3	5	80
Sandwich-type cookies, chocolate or vanilla, 2	4.5	1.2	8	96
Chocolate-frosted cupcake, 1	4.5	1.8	17	121
Frosted cream-filled cupcake, 1	5.2	1.7	26	194
Doughnut, cake-type, 1	6.0	1.5	19	160
Doughnut, raised, 1	11.2	2.8	10	99

Reprinted by permission of Health Information Services, Merck Sharp & Downes, Division of Merck & Co., Inc., West Point, PA 19486, based on material originally developed by the U.S. Department of Agriculture.

FIBER CONTENT OF
HIGH- FIBER FOODS

Fiber in grams

Corn bran	3½ ounces	62
Wheat bran	1 cup	23.8
Cornmeal, whole-grain	1 cup	19.8
Rye flour, dark	1 cup	16.2
Oat flour, whole-grain	3½ ounces	14
Whole wheat	1 cup	13.0
Cornmeal, degermed	1 cup	12.8
Wheat germ	3½ ounces	9.5
Buckwheat groats, cooked	3½ ounces	6.0
Whole-wheat pasta	1 cup	5.4
Oat bran	¼ cup	5.3
Brown rice, cooked	1 cup	4.3
All-Bran with Extra Fiber (Kellogg's)	1 ounce	13.0
Fiber One (General Mills)	1 ounce	12.0
Nabisco 100% Bran	1 ounce	9.1
All-Bran (Kellogg's)	1 ounce	8.6
Bran Buds	1 ounce	7.8
Natural Bran Flakes	1 ounce	5.0
Bran Chex	1 ounce	4.6
Fruit 'n' Fiber	1 ounce	4.0
Shredded Wheat 'n' Bran	1 ounce	4.0
Wheatena	¾ cup	4.5
Oatmeal (Quaker)	¾ cup	2.9
Kidney beans (cooked)	½ cup	9.7
Pinto beans	½ cup	8.9
White beans	½ cup	7.9
Lima beans	½ cup	7.3
Peas (canned)	½ cup	5.3
Baked potato	1 plain	4.8
Corn, sweet	½ cup	4.7
Broccoli (raw)	3½ ounces	4.1
Peas (frozen)	½ cup	4.0

		Fiber in grams
Carrot, cooked	½ cup	2.9
Cabbage, cooked	½ cup	2.1
Raspberries	½ cup	9.2
Mango	1 medium	4.6
Pears	1 medium	4.0
Apple	1 medium	3.2
Banana	1 medium	3.0
Orange	1 medium	2.8

Source: The above information is derived with permission from *The Dietary Fiber Counter to Brand-Name & Whole Foods,* copyright © by Lynn Sonberg, (Berkeley, 1987), edited by Lynn Sonberg. Reprinted by permission. This is an excellent, comprehensive reference that lists the fiber content of virtually every kind of food, both fresh and popular brand-name items—an indispensable guide to healthy eating.

REFERENCES AND GENERAL READING

The Book of Whole Meals by Annemarie Colbin. New York: Ballantine, 1979 and 1983.

Anne Wigmore's Recipes for Longer Life by Anne Wigmore. Wayne, N.J.: Avery Publishing Group, 1978.

The Good Food Compendium by Jo Giese Brown. New York: Doubleday/Dolphin, 1981.

Jane Brody's Nutrition Book by Jane Brody. New York: Bantam, 1981, reissued 1987.

The Pritikin Program for Diet & Exercise by Nathan Pritikin with Patrick McGrady, Jr. New York: Bantam, 1979.

The Macrobiotic Way: The Complete Macrobiotic Diet & Exercise Book by Michio Kushi with Stephen Blauer. Wayne, N.J.: Avery Publishing Group, 1985.

Making the Transition to a Macrobiotic Diet by Carolyn Heidenry. Wayne, N.J.: Avery Publishing Group, 1984.

The Allergy Self-Help Book by Sharon Faelton and the editors of *Prevention* magazine. Emmaus, Pa.: Rodale, 1983.

Coping with Food Allergy by Claude A. Frazier, M.D. New York: Quadrangle, 1985, revised ed.

Wholesome Diet, Library of Health. New York: Time Life Books, 1981.

Goldbeck's Guide to Good Food by Nikki and David Goldbeck. New York: NAL, 1987.

The Complete Eater's Digest and Nutrition Scoreboard by Michael Jacobson, Ph.D. New York: Anchor Press, 1985.

The Fast Food Guide by Michael Jacobson, Ph.D., and Sarah Fritschner. New York: Workman, 1986.

The Dietary Fiber Counter to Brand-Name and Whole Foods, edited by Lynn Sonberg. New York: Berkley, 1987.

Calorie Guide to Brand Names & Basic Foods by Barbara Kraus. New York: Signet, 1985.

INDEX